Acquiring Critical Thinking Skills

Marilyn Meltzer, MA

Hunter College
New York, New York

Susan Marcus Palau, MA

Learning Specialist
Private Practice
Westchester, New York

W.B. SAUNDERS COMPANY

A Division of Harcourt Brace & Company

Philadelphia   London   Toronto
Montreal   Sydney   Tokyo

W.B. SAUNDERS COMPANY

A Division of Harcourt Brace & Company

The Curtis Center
Independence Square West
Philadelphia, PA 19106

Library of Congress Cataloging–in–Publication Data

Meltzer, Marilyn
    Acquiring critical thinking skills / Marilyn Meltzer, Susan Marcus
Palau.
      p.   cm.
    ISBN 0–7216–6151–3
    1. Nursing—Study and teaching. 2. Critical thinking.   3. Study
skills. I. Palau, Susan Marcus. II. Title.
RT73.M394 1996
610. 73'071—dc20

95–42974

ACQUIRING CRITICAL THINKING SKILLS

ISBN 0–7216–6151–3

Printed in the United States of America

Last digit is the print number: 9 8 7 6 5 4 3 2 1

For Joe Palau, PhD,
husband and philosopher

For Sheldon, Sara, and Michael

Preface

Acquiring Critical Thinking Skills is intended for students in the allied health fields who need to learn how to apply problem-solving strategies to their school and work assignments.

Among the employment requisites for the twenty-first century will be the ability to apply the information and skills learned in school to job tasks. The purpose of this text is to teach students the critical thinking skills in reading, writing, mathematics, and studying that will help them solve problems in their courses or their work in the health fields. Many of the exercises use material taken from recent textbooks in health fields so that students can practice applying these critical thinking skills in the actual context of their chosen field.

▼ ORGANIZATION

Unit I, Applying Critical Thinking Skills to Reading, will help students become active readers by improving their abilities to understand, interpret, apply, and evaluate the information they read.

Unit II, Applying Critical Thinking Skills to Writing, will help students learn how to plan, organize, and evaluate information so that they can produce clear, logical writing in school or at work.

Unit III, Applying Critical Thinking Skills to Mathematics, will help students learn the processes and strategies needed for accurate solutions in their computations, conversions, and problem solving.

Unit IV, Applying Critical Thinking Skills to Studying, will help students learn how to assess and improve their study techniques.

Each chapter in Units I through IV includes the following features:

- Objectives: Learning Objectives are presented.
- Vocabulary: In this method of vocabulary study the students identify vocabulary words, predict meanings, apply definitions, evaluate definitions, and make necessary revisions. As a preview strategy, students are asked to find words in the chapter whose meanings are unclear to them. They are asked to use background knowledge to predict the definition of each word. They are also asked to use the word in a sentence. After they have read the chapter, the students are asked to evaluate the correctness of their use of

each word in a sentence. If they use any word incorrectly, they are asked to revise their sentences.

- Introduction of critical thinking skills: Critical thinking skills are introduced through the use of examples and practice exercises. Each chapter introduces the following critical thinking skills:
  - *Understanding* gives students practice in recalling and comprehending information.
  - *Interpreting* helps students learn to analyze and synthesize information.
  - *Applying* helps students learn how to use their newly acquired information in a practical or theoretical way.
  - *Evaluating* helps students learn how to judge, rate, or measure what they have learned.
- Critical Reading: The students are asked to read a selection from a health care textbook and to apply active reading skills by using the previewing, questioning, applying, and evaluating strategies that they are learning.
- Student Journal: The journal at the end of each chapter gives students an opportunity to reflect on what they have learned in the chapter and on how these strategies can be used to improve study or work in the health fields. Journal writing encourages critical thinking about information that has been learned.

▼ USING THE TEXTBOOK

Acquiring Critical Thinking Skills is designed to be used in one semester. One chapter can be completed each week during a 15-week semester. This text can be used in conjunction with or as a sequel to *Learning Strategies for Allied Health Students* by Palau and Meltzer. The two texts together can be used in a 30-week, two-semester course.

▼ SETTING UP THE COURSE

Acquiring Critical Thinking Skills can be used in a classroom setting with the instructor providing guided practice, or students can use this book independently as a study resource. The text is divided into four units, which can be used in any order. The instructor can evaluate students' work, or students can assess their own progress by using the Answer Key at the back of the book. Students can be encouraged to work collaboratively in small groups or individually at their own pace.

▼ ACKNOWLEDGMENTS

We would like to thank Lisa Biello and Suzanne Hontscharik of W.B. Saunders, who helped in the preparation of the manuscript, and Mary Espenschied of CRACOM Corporation, who helped in the production process.

Thank you to Sara Meltzer and Michael Meltzer for their word-processing talents, Joe Palau for his philosophical insights, Agnes Sinko, Director of the Irvington Public Library, for her research assistance, and our students, who are always our inspiration.

Marilyn Meltzer
Susan Marcus Palau

Contents

UNIT I ●

Applying Critical Thinking Skills to Reading

Applying critical thinking skills to reading will help you to understand your text-books and to perform successfully in your work in the health fields.

Unit I will help you to learn to apply these critical thinking skills to your reading assignments in school and at work.

Chapter 1, Defining the Terminology, teaches the importance of learning accurate meanings for words from your health care textbooks and how to apply these meanings to improve your reading comprehension. Chapter 2, Differentiating Fact from Opinion, helps you to learn how to differentiate fact from opinion in your readings and to avoid acting on opinions as if they were facts. Chapter 3, Detecting Biases, shows you how to detect biases in your readings, personal life, and the workplace. Chapter 4, Making Value Judgments from Readings, teaches you to make value judgments based on fact and to avoid allowing emotionally charged words to influence your ability to make value judgments. In Chapter 5, Resolving Conflicts, you will learn how to analyze conflicts and find appropriate solutions.

The chapters in Unit I will provide you with the critical thinking skills needed to improve your comprehension of reading texts and to fulfill reading tasks more successfully in the workplace.

Chapter 1

Defining the Terminology

▼ LEARNING OBJECTIVES

In this chapter you learn how to

- Learn accurate meanings for words from your health care texts
- Apply these meanings to help you understand the reading selection

▼ PREDICTING VOCABULARY

Directions: Preview this chapter by finding 5 words that you recognize but whose precise definition you don't know. Use your background knowledge to write a sentence for each word that predicts the definition of that word.

Word 1: _____

Sentence: _____

_____

Word 2: _____

Sentence: _____

_____

Word 3: _____

Sentence: _____

_____

Word 4: _____

Sentence: _____

_____

Word 5: _____

Sentence: _____

_____

When you finish reading this chapter, evaluate the accuracy of your sentences. Make any necessary revisions.

Revisions

_____

_____

_____

_____

_____

_____

_____

_____

▼ UNDERSTANDING DEFINING THE TERMINOLOGY

As a reader you come across words whose meanings you vaguely understand. Using context clues helps you to approximate the definition of the word. When you are reading fiction or text in certain subject areas, meanings that are almost correct may be enough to help you understand the ideas in the passage. However, in the health fields, imprecise meanings are not enough. Unless you know the precise definitions of words, you can make mistakes in your reading. Even worse, you can make errors when you attempt to apply the information from your reading to your work in the health fields. To find precise definitions of unfamiliar words, get in the habit of looking up word meanings in a glossary (a dictionary of key words, found in most textbooks) or a medical dictionary.

Example 1–1

Read the following two sentences. Then read how knowing the precise meaning of each word affects your comprehension of the sentence.

1. Some infants are fed with breast milk and some are fed with commercially prepared formula.

In this sentence *formula* means a milk mixture that is fed to babies. It does not mean the rules for a mathematical equation.

2. Doctors do not always agree on when babies should begin eating solid food.

In this sentence the precise meaning of solid is the opposite of liquid. It does not mean hard. Feeding an infant hard food would be dangerous.

Directions: Read the following 10 sentences. Write the precise definition of each italicized word. If you don't know the precise definition, look up the meaning of the word in a medical dictionary. Notice how knowing the precise word meaning affects your comprehension of the sentence.

1. The trauma to the *cranial* cavity was a lasting head injury.

   _____

2. The *pelvic* cavity had a collection of inflammatory fluid.

   _____

3. There was a rupture in his *diaphragm.*

   _____

4. The cancer spread to her *spinal column* and caused her severe back pain.

   _____

5. The singer had an infection in her *larynx.*

   _____

6. Food was stuck in her *pharynx* and caused her to choke.

   _____

7. He tore the *cartilage* in his knee while he was playing tennis.

   _____

8. The blockage in his *trachea* caused breathing problems.

   _____

9. The *genes* are responsible for eye color.

   _____

10. A slowdown in *metabolism* can cause weight gain.

   _____

Another way for you to become familiar with health care terms and their meanings is to learn the following word parts:

- *roots* (bases of words)
- *prefixes* (beginnings of words that change word meanings)
- *suffixes* (word endings)

Become familiar with the following lists of prefixes, roots, and suffixes and their meanings from *The Language of Medicine* (Chabner, pp. 10, 13, and 17). Many of these word parts are medical terms.

Example 1–2

Prefix	Meaning	Root	Meaning	Suffix	Meaning
endo	within	arthr	joint	al	pertaining to
epi	above,	bio	life	cyte	cell
	beyond	cardi	heart	ectomy	removal
ex	out	cephal	head	genic	process
hyper	excessive,	cis	to cut	ist	specialist
	above	gastr	stomach	itis	inflammation
hypo	deficient,	gynec	woman,	logy	study of
	below		female	pathy	disease
in	in, into	hemat	blood		condition
peri	surrounding	neur	nerve	scope	instrument
pro	before	oste	bone		to visually
re	back				examine
sub	below,			tomy	process of
	under				cutting into

The word *exocardial* can be divided into the following word parts:
The **prefix** *ex* means out.
The **root** *cardi* means heart.
The **suffix** *al* means pertaining to.
Exocardial means pertaining to outside the heart.

Directions: Use the list of prefix, suffix, and root meanings in Example 1–2 to write the definition of the following medical terms.

1. Hypertension _____

2. Hyperthyroid _____

3. Hypodermic _____

4. Urologist _____

5. Hematology _____

6. Prognosis _____

7. Neurology _____

8. Resection _____

9. Gynecology _____

10. Incision _____

When you are reading longer selections, be aware of words whose precise meaning you do not know. Learning these meanings will help you to understand the ideas in the selection.

Example 1–3

Read the following selection from *The Language of Medicine* (Chabner, p. 566). Pay attention to the boldface words and the precise definitions given for these words. Think about how knowing these definitions helped you to understand the passage.

Acne **vulgaris** (**vulgaris** means ordinary) is caused by the build up of sebum and keratin in the pores of the skin. A **blackhead** or **comedo** (plural: **comedones**) is a sebum plug partially blocking the pore. If the pore becomes completely blocked, a **whitehead** forms. Bacteria in the skin break down the sebum, producing inflammation in the surrounding tissue. Papules, pustules, and cysts can thus form. Treatment consists of long-term antibiotic use and medications to dry the skin. Benzoyl peroxide and tretinoin (Retin-A) are medications to prevent comedo formation; isotretinoin (Accutane) is used in severe cystic acne.

Directions: Read the following selection from *The Language of Medicine* (Chabner, p. 567). Write the precise meaning of the boldface words. Then write how learning these word meanings helped you to understand the passage.

1–4

PSORIASIS

Chronic, recurrent dermatosis marked by itchy, scaly, red patches covered by silvery gray scales.

Psoriasis commonly forms on the forearms, knees, legs, and scalp. It is neither infectious nor contagious, but it is caused by an increased rate of growth of the basal layer of the epidermis. Etiology is unknown, but the condition runs in families and may be brought on by anxiety. Treatment is palliative (relieving but not curing) with topical lubricants, keratolytics, and steroids. **PUVA** (psoralen–ultraviolet A light therapy) is also used.

1. Psoriasis means _____.

2. PUVA means _____.

3. These precise definitions helped me to understand the meaning of the

   passage because _____.

▼ INTERPRETING DEFINING THE TERMINOLOGY

When you are reading a selection in a health care text, knowing precise word meanings will help you to comprehend the technical information in the selection. Once you know the exact word meanings, you are ready to interpret the author's information.

Example 1–4

Read the following selection from *The Language of Medicine* (Chabner, p. 723). Notice how learning the precise definition of **fluoroscopy** helps you to interpret the advantage of using fluoroscopy over normal radiography.

Fluoroscopy. This x-ray procedure uses a fluorescent screen instead of a photographic plate to derive a visual image from the x-rays that pass through the patient. The fact that ionizing radiation such as x-rays can produce fluorescence (rays of light energy emitted as a result of exposure to and absorption of radiation from another source) is the basis for fluoroscopy. The fluorescent screen glows when it is struck by the x-rays. Opaque tissue, such as bone, appears as a dark shadow image on the fluorescent screen.

A major advantage of fluoroscopy over normal radiography is that internal organs, such as the heart and digestive tract organs, can be observed in motion. Also, the patient's position can be changed constantly to provide the right view at the right time so that the most useful diagnostic information can be obtained.

EXERCISE
1–5

Directions: Read the following selection from *The Language of Medicine* (Chabner, p. 729) and answer the questions below. Notice how knowing the precise definitions of the words in boldface type helps you to understand the information in the selection.

Nuclear medicine physicians use two types of tests in the diagnosis of disease: **in vitro** (in the test tube) procedures and **in vivo** (in the body) procedures. **In vitro** procedures involve analysis of blood and urine specimens using radioactive chemicals. For example, a **radioimmunoassay (RIA)** is an in vitro procedure that combines the use of radioactive chemicals and antibodies to detect hormones and drugs in a patient's blood. The test allows the detection of minute amounts of drug. RIA is used to monitor the amount of digitalis, a drug used to treat heart disease, in a patient's bloodstream and can detect hypothyroidism in newborn infants.

In vivo tests trace the amounts of radioactive substances within the body. They are given directly to a patient to evaluate the function of an organ or to image it. For example, in **tracer studies** a specific radionuclide is incorporated into a chemical substance and administered to a patient. The combination of the radionuclide and a drug or chemical is called a **radiopharmaceutical** (or **labeled compound**). Each radiopharmaceutical is designed to concentrate in a certain organ. The organ can then be imaged with the radiation given off by the radionuclide.

1. What is the difference between **in vitro** and **in vivo** procedures? _____

   _____

2. How can an organ be imaged? _____

   _____

3. How do tracer studies work? _____

   _____

4. Why is RIA useful? _____

   _____

5. How is nuclear medicine helping physicians diagnose disease? _____

   _____

▼ APPLYING DEFINING THE TERMINOLOGY

It is important for you to know the precise meanings of words when you have to carry out tasks in the workplace.

Example 1–5

Read the following selection from *Computer Concepts and Applications for the Medical Office* (Bonewit-West, p. 91). Notice how learning the precise definition of text formatting will help you to arrange the information on the printed page.

Formatting Text

Text formatting is the arrangement or layout of the text on paper; in other words, how it will appear as printed text. Text entering and printing are two separate functions in word processing. This is in contrast to the typewriter in which these functions occur simultaneously, and the format is integrated as the document is being typed. Because of this separation in word processing, a document can be formatted a number of different ways by simply changing the formatting instructions. For example, if a document has been printed using single spacing, and the user desires the same document in a double-spaced format, the line spacing value can be changed from single- to double-spacing without having to retype the document. Formatting options included in most word processing programs are listed and described on the following page.

Directions: Read the following selection from *Computer Concepts and Applications for the Medical Office* (Bonewit-West, p. 138). Answer the following questions.

EXERCISE 1–6

Types of Start-Up Tasks

Start-up tasks require the entering of data that is used on a daily basis into your computer. This data then becomes part of the medical practice database and is organized in a manner which allows for later retrieval and use. The specific start-up tasks that must be performed to make the computer system operational are listed and briefly described below.

Practice Information: This start-up task customizes your computer system with the name, address, phone number and federal tax identification number of your medical practice.

User Passwords: This start-up task provides security to your computer system by assigning a password to each individual using the computer. This password must be typed in by the user before he/she can work on the computer.

Providers: This start-up task allows you to enter and store information regarding the physicians in your medical practice. As a result, anytime this information is needed on a document or form (e.g., insurance claim form) the computer system will transfer this information from the provider file and place it on the form.

Diagnosis Codes: This start-up task lets you compile and store a list of diagnoses along with their corresponding ICD-9-CM codes. This information can then be transferred to any document requiring it such as superbills and insurance claim forms.

Procedure Codes: This start-up task allows you to compile and store a list of medical services and procedures performed in your medical office along with the CPT-4 code and standard office charge for each procedure. This information can then be transferred to any document requiring it.

Insurance Carriers: An *insurance carrier* is a company that provides an insurance policy. Other names for an insurance carrier include: insurer, third-party carrier and third-party payor. This start-up task allows you to enter and store information regarding the insurance carriers used by patients in the practice which is needed for processing insurance claims.

Place of Service: This start-up task allows you to compile and store information on the facilities where the physician performs medical services and procedures.

Referring Physicians: This start-up task lets you compile and store information about physicians who refer patients to your medical office.

1. Which start-up task enables you to provide security to your computer system? _____

_____

2. Which start-up task allows you to store information on where the physician performs medical services? _____

_____

3. Who are the providers? _____

_____

4. Why do you need to store information on insurance carriers? _____

_____

_____

5. What would happen if you confused the meanings of diagnosis codes and procedure codes? _____

_____

_____

▼ EVALUATING DEFINING THE TERMINOLOGY

In your studies or work in the health care fields, you will have to make decisions. If you do not know the precise meaning of a word in a reading selection or set of directions, you could make errors that would have negative effects on your studies or your career.

Example 1–6

Read the following selection from *EMT Prehospital Care* (Henry and Stapleton, p. 308). Notice how knowing that the word **deteriorating** means worsening can help you make a decision on the seriousness of a head injury.

Signs of Increased Intracranial Pressure

As pressure within the cranium rises, certain signs and symptoms appear. The conscious patient may complain of *headaches, nausea, and vomiting*. Sometimes the vomiting is *projectile*, meaning that the vomitus is ejected from the mouth with considerable force.

The *level of consciousness may begin to deteriorate*. The patient who was previously alert now gets sleepy or more confused and is more difficult to arouse. Instead of responding to verbal commands, the patient may eventually respond to painful stimuli only.

Children are more likely to experience drowsiness and nausea and vomiting after even minor head injuries. The seriousness of these signs can be determined only after a careful neurologic examination. In the field the EMT must regard these signs as possible indications of increasing intracranial pressure.

The most sensitive indicator of increasing intracranial pressure is a changing (deteriorating) level of consciousness. After suffering a head injury, the damage due to the direct blow—concussion or contusion or disruption of the blood supply—has been completed. Signs present immediately following the injury can be attributed to the blow itself.

Any worsening of the condition can no longer be explained as due to the initial impact but must be considered the result of secondary forces—such as increased intracranial pressure from bleeding or swelling within the skull. This is especially the case if there are no other complications such as hypoxia or hypotension to explain the deterioration in status.

Directions: Read the following selection from *EMT Prehospital Care* (Henry and Stapleton, p. 45) and answer the questions that follow based on the precise definitions of the italicized words.

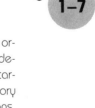

EXERCISE 1-7

Heart. Tracing the need for oxygen demonstrates the most dramatic example of the organ systems' interdependence. The brain can only function for 10 seconds or less if deprived of all oxygen. If the heart stops and circulation of blood to the brain ceases (cardiac arrest), consciousness is lost within 10 seconds, and shortly thereafter all respiratory effort ceases. Lack of oxygen flow to the brain, as evidenced by no pulse and respirations, causes the condition known as *clinical death*. If the brain is deprived of oxygen for 4 to 6 minutes, *biological death* begins. Biological death defines a state of sustained oxygen deprivation after which recovery without brain damage is unlikely.

The time to biological death is modified by certain factors or conditions. For example, children have greater tolerance for sustained pulselessness than do adults. A cool body temperature lowers the body's metabolism and improves the chances of recovery. Drowning often arouses reflexes (e.g., the mammalian diving reflex—a reaction to cold water that shuts off major blood flow throughout the body, except to the brain, heart, and lungs) that improve the chances of recovery as well.

1. Clinical death means _____

2. Biological death means _____

3. Which would most likely cause brain damage? How would the knowledge of the differences between these terms affect decisions of a physician?

_____

_____

_____

CRITICAL READING

Previewing

Preview this selection. Think about what you already know concerning this topic. In the space provided, write what you still wish to know.

_____

_____

_____

_____

_____

_____

Questioning

Based on your preview, formulate questions that will help you learn what you still wish to know about the topic.

_____

_____

_____

_____

_____

_____

Reading

Read the following selection from *Saunders Fundamentals for Nursing* (Polaski and Warner, pp. 515-517):

Sensory Deprivation

Sensory deprivation is the condition of inadequate stimulation, in terms of both quality (type of stimulation) and quantity (amount of stimulation). Sensory deprivation can be caused by an environmental situation such as a room with colorless walls; dim lights; and no windows, pictures, calendars, or books. Life becomes dull without the stimulation of all the senses.

Sensory deprivation can also be caused by the patient's condition. Patients who are in an isolation room because of infection or who cannot move because of a cast may be deprived of the sensory stimulation they normally enjoy. Deprivation can also be caused by a deficit of one of the five senses. In this case, because patients cannot receive stimuli, they are deprived of normal, healthy stimulation of the senses.

Another reason sensory deprivation may occur is that a patient is not able to process (use) stimuli. This means that although sensory organs receive stimulation, they are not able to understand or interpret the stimuli in the usual way. Diseases that affect the brain (for example, stroke and cancer) can interfere with the ability to process stimuli. In diseases that cause necrosis (death of tissue) in the brain, the affected part of the brain can no longer receive and interpret sensory information.

Drugs that depress brain function, such as alcohol and narcotics, can also interfere with the person's ability to process incoming stimuli. When alcohol is present in the body, it decreases the function of the brain. It does not send messages to the body as quickly as usual.

Finally, sensory deprivation can result if there is a language barrier. The patient may not be able to understand information without the help of an interpreter. They can hear when spoken to, but do not understand what is said because of a lack of knowledge of that specific language.

Observations of the Patient with Sensory Deprivation. The patient who experiences sensory deprivation may exhibit a variety of behaviors. It may be difficult to communicate with this patient. Ask simple questions about usual events in the patient's life. Observe for fatigue, boredom, and decreased interest in surroundings. The deprivation may cause the patient to have a poor appetite or sleeping problems such as **insomnia** or restlessness. Patients may tell you they have physical discomforts (for example, headache or stomachache) that are unexplained. Sensory deprivation is most notable in patients who are in the intensive care unit. Think about the dull, sterile environment of the special care units found in the hospital.

Care of the Patient with Sensory Deprivation. You need to provide patients who have sensory deprivation with the sensory stimulation that is missing. For example, to give the patient a sense of the time of day, you can

- Use less lighting during the night.
- Put day clothing on the patient during the day and night clothes on at night whenever possible.
- Keep a calendar or clock in the room to help orient the patient to time.
- While you are giving care, mention the time of the day, week, or month to the patient.
- Mention any changes in the seasons.

To provide other sensory stimulation, you can

- Sit the patient in a chair by the window for visual stimulation.
- Use color and activity to stimulate the patient's senses.
- Provide music during the day for auditory stimulation. You should ask a family member about the patient's preference in music.
- Encourage visitors to add stimulation to the environment by their presence and efforts to talk with the patient.

SENSORY DEPRIVATION
a condition in which a person receives less than normal sensory input; there is inadequate quality or quantity of stimuli

INSOMNIA
the inability to fall asleep easily or remain asleep throughout the night

Seizure Disorder, a Disruption in Sensory Function

SEIZURE

a change in body function caused by abnormal electrical activity in the brain; convulsion

AURA

an odd feeling, such as numbness or dizziness, just before a seizure or migraine headache starts

A **seizure** is a change in body function caused by abnormal electrical activity in the brain. A seizure is also known as a convulsion. There are many different types of seizures. A person who experiences any type of seizure is said to have a seizure disorder. If your patient has a history of seizure disorder, you will be notified of this when you receive a report from the nurse or your supervisor before you give care.

You should observe for the following:

- patient reports of an **aura**
- sudden stiffening of the limbs
- jerking movements of the limbs
- changes in consciousness, such as appearing to daydream or the inability to respond to commands
- eye changes such as
    Turning of the eye and head to one side or the other
    Changes in the size of pupils
- other changes may include
    An increase in saliva
    Tongue or lip biting
    Incontinence of bowel or bladder
    Changes in the breathing pattern, such as appearing to stop breathing

Each person responds to a seizure disorder differently. You will not observe all of the changes listed above in all patients with seizure disorders. This list just gives the changes most commonly observed. Many other changes might occur, depending on the part of the brain that is affected. Observe for anything different from the usual.

A person is at high risk for injury during a seizure. As a nursing assistant, you should be familiar with the seizure precaution policy in your health care institution. If a seizure occurs, you should

- Note the time the seizure began.
- Turn patients on their side, if possible.
- Support the head with a pillow.
- Call for help by turning on the call signal:
    The nurse may need to use suction equipment if saliva closes off air supply to the lungs.
    The nurse may decide to give oxygen.
- Stay with the patient and observe for any changes.
- Note the time the seizure ends.

After the seizure is over, the patient may

- Be difficult to wake up.
- Be unaware that a seizure occurred.
- Feel sleepy and sleep for several hours.

You should make the patient comfortable and make the room quiet and comfortable for sleep. After the seizure is over, report and record your observations.

In recent years, the focus of caring for the patient with seizure disorder has changed. The focus now is on keeping the patient safe. Follow these guidelines to keep patients safe during a seizure.

- *Never place a padded tongue blade between the teeth.* During a seizure, the jaws tighten. Forcing a tongue blade between the teeth can chip the enamel and place the patient at risk for breathing the pieces into the lungs.
- Padded side rails are not encouraged because of the embarrassment they may cause the patient and family.
- If patients are doing something active when the seizure occurs, you may need to help them lie down in a safe place.

Sensory Overload

Sensory overload occurs when a person receives an excessive amount of sensory stimulation. It is generally more stimulation than can be tolerated by the individual within a given time period. The brain reacts to the sensory overload by not responding appropriately. You are responsible for observing the behavior of a patient who may have sensory overload. The response to sensory stimulation is very individualized.

Observation of the Patient with Sensory Overload. The patient with sensory overload may display nervous or anxious behaviors (for example, irritability or crying). You may notice that the patient who tires easily may have disturbed sleep. Too much stimulation for the brain to interpret may cause a change in appetite. The patient may have no desire to eat and may just move the food around until it is taken away. In sensory overload, the brain cannot concentrate and you will observe a short attention span.

Care of the Patient with Sensory Overload. Whenever there is an overabundance (too much) of stimulation, you need to change the environment to block the incoming stimulation. The following are some measures you can take to help decrease stimuli in the patient's environment.

- Reduce bright lights and eliminate extra movement in the surroundings.
- Place a folded washcloth over patients' eyes to lessen visual overstimulation.
- Decrease offensive noises in the environment.
- Encourage the patient to listen to soft music through a set of earphones.
- Remember that patients with sensory overload may need help interpreting information and understanding it.
- Explain to patients what you are doing and what is happening around them.
- Use simple words and short sentences.
- Ask patients to take deep breaths and imagine themselves in a quiet place.
- Whenever possible, reduce any stimulation that is more than patients can handle.

SENSORY OVERLOAD
a condition in which a person receives too many stimuli to the senses

Applying

In the space provided answer your questions.

_____

_____

_____

_____

_____

_____

_____

_____

_____

_____

_____

Evaluating

Were you able to answer all your questions? Yes _____ No _____. Did the selection give you enough information about the topic? Explain.

_____

_____

_____

_____

_____

_____

_____

_____

_____

_____

Check the accuracy of your answers by locating the specific information in the selection.

STUDENT JOURNAL

List what you have learned about defining the terminology.	How would you apply this knowledge to your study or work in the health fields?

Chapter 2

Differentiating Fact from Opinion

▼ LEARNING OBJECTIVES

In this chapter you will learn how to
- Differentiate fact from opinion in your readings
- Avoid acting on opinions as if they were facts

▼ PREDICTING VOCABULARY

Directions: Preview this chapter by finding five words that you recognize but whose precise definition you don't know. Use your background knowledge to write a sentence for each word that predicts the definition of that word.

Word 1: _____

Sentence: _____

_____

Word 2: _____

Sentence: _____

_____

Word 3: _____

Sentence: _____

_____

Word 4: _____

Sentence: _____

_____

Word 5: _____

Sentence: _____

_____

When you finish reading this chapter, evaluate the accuracy of your sentences. Make any necessary revisions.

Revisions

_____

_____

_____

_____

_____

_____

_____

_____

▼ UNDERSTANDING DIFFERENTIATING FACT FROM OPINION

Many readers have difficulty differentiating between fact and opinion. A fact can be proved. An opinion cannot be proved; an opinion is someone's belief. When you are reading, you must be able to distinguish fact from opinion. To avoid confusing fact and opinion, learn to check information against the criteria for facts and the criteria for opinions.

Check Test for Facts
A **fact** is

- objective, free from prejudice in judgment
- something that can be observed or measured
- verified by testing, research, or experimentation

Check Test for Opinions
An **opinion** is

- subjective, based on individual judgment
- suggested by clue words such as
  - in my opinion
  - without doubt
  - I believe
  - claims

Many readers mistake opinions for facts. Acting on opinions as if they were facts leads to errors in thinking and problem solving.

One reason readers accept opinions as facts is that they agree with the opinions. Readers should be aware of their own **bias,** a prejudice for or against something, when they examine information. Do not allow your subjective feelings to influence your judgment when reading. Differentiating fact from opinion will enable you to be a better critical reader and thinker.

Example 2–1

Let's read the following sentences and apply the check test for facts.

1. Many household cleaning solutions are poisonous when swallowed.
   Is this sentence
   a. objective? _Yes_ .
   b. something that can be observed or measured? _Yes_ .
   c. something that can be verified by testing, research, or experimentation? _Yes_ .
2. Toddlers think that medication is candy.
   Is this sentence
   a. objective? _No_ , it implies someone's feelings about toddlers.
   b. something that can be observed or measured? _No_ , you cannot see someone "think."
   c. something that can be verified by testing, research, or experimentation? _No_ , you cannot test someone's thoughts objectively.

Therefore sentence 1 is a fact and sentence 2 is opinion.

EXERCISE 2–2

Directions: Read the following sentences. Next to each sentence, write whether it is a fact or an opinion. As you read each sentence, apply the check test for facts and opinions.

_____ 1. Preschool children prefer riding a tricycle to walking.

_____ 2. Rhubarb leaves are poisonous.

_____ 3. Contaminated food can cause illness.

_____ 4. Matches are more dangerous to preschool children than is hot coffee.

_____ 5. Exposed wires are dangerous.

_____ 6. A toddler is older than an infant.

_____ 7. A toddler faces more unsafe situations than an infant.

_____ 8. Poisonous liquids can cause death.

_____ 9. Children are afraid of wet floors.

_____10. Wet floors are a source of accidents.

Example 2–2

Read the following selection from *Saunders Fundamentals for Nursing Assistants* (Polaski and Warner, p. 268). Then read the question and answer that follow to further your understanding of differentiating fact from opinion in a reading selection.

Safety

Safety is the condition of being free from experiencing or causing hurt, injury, or loss. Everyone has a need for safety. Your patients stay safe because of measures you take to limit or prevent hurt, injury, or loss. Safety practices are important for your safety as well. Common activities that keep a person safe are

- not walking across wet floors because a fall could result in injury
- keeping foods refrigerated to prevent the growth of harmful **microorganisms** in certain foods. When the contaminated (spoiled) food is eaten, illness may occur
- checking electrical cords for frayed cords or exposed wires
- helping small children or weak elderly persons down steps because you know they cannot manage walking down stairs alone

Many daily safety activities are performed automatically. Part of the comfort of your own home is created by the safety practices you perform for yourself and those you love, for example, keeping sharp knives in a safe place. In the health care institution, you use many of these safety activities and learn others to create a safe **environment** for yourself and your patients. You need to learn about the safety needs of people of all ages. You are responsible for keeping patients and their environment safe so that no one is hurt or injured.

Question: What four facts mentioned in this passage could prevent harm to members of your household?

Answer: Common activities that promote a safe environment are (1) not allowing members to walk on wet floors in order to prevent falls, (2) keeping foods refrigerated to prevent illness from spoiled food, (3) checking frayed cords or exposed wires to prevent burns and shock, and (4) helping young children and older family members walk down stairs to prevent falls.

SAFETY
the status of being safe from experiencing or causing hurt, injury, or loss

MICROORGANISM
an organism so tiny it can be seen only under a microscope; capable of helping the body as well as causing disease

ENVIRONMENT
the conditions, circumstances, or objects that surround a person

---

Directions: Read the following selection from *Saunders Fundamentals for Nursing Assistants* (Polaski and Warner, pp. 268-270). Answer the question that follows to check your understanding of how to differentiate fact from opinion in a reading selection.

EXERCISE 2-3

Safety for Infants and Toddlers

Infants and **toddlers** need a safe environment in which to thrive. Infants and toddlers are too young to use the **problem-solving process** to save themselves from harm. Therefore, adults (the parents or care giver) must create a safe environment for them. In this age group (from birth to about 3 years), children face many unsafe and potentially life-threatening situations. Accidents often occur because parents mistakenly think the infant can or cannot do something.

INFANT
the person at the beginning of life (from birth to 1½ years), for whom all needs are met by others

TODDLER
the child from 1½ to 3 years of age

PROBLEM-SOLVING PROCESS
the systematic method used to resolve problems

Typical Accidents

Falls. Infants who are learning to roll over are interested in the "how" of rolling. They are not aware that they are on a changing table, crib, bed, or couch and can roll off. Infants and toddlers do not like to be restricted in their movement and try to climb out of high chairs, walkers, and cribs without realizing the potential for a fall. Infants and toddlers can injure themselves if they are carrying a sharp object or a broken toy when they fall. Falls may result in broken bones or head injuries.

Burns. Infants do not fully understand the concepts of hot and cold. The handle of a pot on the stove looks inviting to them. They may pull it down and spill hot food or fluids on themselves, resulting in a serious burn. Infants and toddlers see extension cords, cigarettes, burning candles, and **humidifiers** (because they are noisy and steamy) as items worthy of investigation.

HUMIDIFIER
a device (run by electricity) that produces a fine mist of water particles

SUFFOCATION
a stop in breathing due to a lack of oxygen

Suffocation. **Suffocation** occurs when an object does not allow air to enter the lungs. A common item like a plastic bag pulled down over the head can block the entry of air into the lungs and cause death. Infants and toddlers love to snuggle into soft things, such as pillows, which can block the entry of air. A small amount of water in a bathtub or a puddle can also block the entry of air and cause accidental death by drowning. The risk of suffocation is also high for the infant who is in a bed with a sleeping adult.

ASPIRATION
the act of inhaling vomitus, mucus, or a small object into the respiratory system; may occur in persons who are unconscious, are under the effects of general anesthesia, or have difficulty swallowing

POISONING
a condition produced by swallowing or breathing in a harmful substance; may also be produced by injection by a stinging insect

Aspiration. Infants and toddlers love to explore by putting objects in their mouths. A small object like a peanut may be breathed into the air passages and block the entry of air into a part of the lungs. A whole hot dog given to an infant or toddler to munch on is dangerous because, if swallowed, it can block the air passages so completely that no air gets to the lungs. Infants and toddlers should have toys that are appropriate to their age. Any small objects, especially toys with small parts, should not be given to them.

Poisoning. Infants and toddlers are busy exploring their surroundings and often get into things that can cause them harm. Colorful pills may look like candy. Harmful fluids may look like soda pop or juice to these age groups, especially if packaged in a similar-shaped bottle. If these substances are swallowed, a child could become seriously ill or even die if not treated quickly and properly. Make sure harmful fluids are kept out of reach to prevent accidental poisoning.

Motor Vehicle Accidents. The best safety practice, now required by law in many states, is the use of safety car seats for all infants, toddlers, and young children. Infants and toddlers like to move around. While exploring, they quickly learn how to unbuckle the belts. This creates an unsafe situation. Accidents can also occur when children crawl or walk unattended in areas (such as roads, driveways, and alleys) where moving vehicles can cause serious injury or loss of life.

List six types of typical accidents for infants and children. Next to each type list one fact given as an example.

_____

_____

_____

_____

_____

_____

▼ INTERPRETING DIFFERENTIATING FACT FROM OPINION

Writers often support their beliefs, or opinions, with facts. If you are reading an author's opinion, check to see if the opinion is supported by verifiable facts. Remember, even if the supporting facts are proved to be true, the author's belief is still an opinion.

Example 2–3

Read the following selection. The author's opinion has been underlined. Notice how each of the italicized facts supports the author's opinion.

<u>If parents supervised their young children more carefully, childhood injuries would be reduced.</u> Infants who are left alone injure themselves when they *fall out* of *high chairs* or *cribs*. Young children left alone in the kitchen can *burn* themselves by touching a *hot pot*. Another common *injury* to young children occurs when they reach into the medicine cabinet and *swallow pills* or other *medications*. Parents have to watch young children closely to protect them from *harm*.

Directions: Read the following selection from *Saunders Fundamentals for Nursing Assistants* (Polaski and Warner, p. 275). Find the facts supporting the opinion that school-age children could be at greater risk of harm than children in younger age groups.

EXERCISE 2–4

Safety for School-Age Children

From ages 6 to 12, children's motor coordination continues to develop. Problem-solving and decision-making skills continue to increase as school-age children learn to cope with the world at home and at school. Physical, active play is common for school-age boys and girls, including running, jumping, swimming, and other sports that sharpen the competitive spirit. Many of the safety concerns for school-age children are the same as for children in younger age groups, including falls, burns, drowning, and motor vehicle accidents. However, school-age children take more control of their behavior and might be tempted to do things or go places that their parents might disapprove of; this could increase the risk of harm.

Typical Accidents

Falls. Because school-age children are so quick and curious and like to test their strength, many falls result in what are known as sports injuries. Sports injuries affect the muscles and bones used in competitive and close-contact sports.

Burns. Children between the ages 6 and 12 are still attracted to fire. They are able to manipulate (handle) small objects quite well and may strike a match or light a lighter just to watch the flame. They want to be able to control the length of time the flame lasts.

SCHOOL-AGE
the child from 6 to 12 years of age (the years before adolescence)

Drowning. As with the younger age groups, drowning may occur in the school-age child. Children this age still need to be supervised when they are near water.

Motor Vehicle Accidents. Remember that children are competitive at this age. They may run out into traffic from between two cars. Children may also ride a bicycle or skateboard or glide on roller skates into traffic. Wheelchair races are a common attraction and a release from boredom in a health care institution.

Personal Safety. Children who are ill may not have control over their environment. There are many unfamiliar people in a health care institution. Many children are trusting, and because they are in a health care institution they may go with any person who comes into the room with a wheelchair or **gurney.** Children could be in danger if they leave their room with anyone who is not associated with the health care institution.

GURNEY

a cart used to transfer patients

▼ APPLYING DIFFERENTIATING FACT FROM OPINION

Remember, problems occur when you act on opinions as if they were facts; therefore it is important for you to distinguish fact from opinion when you apply the information you are reading.

For example, a health care worker reads an article expressing the opinion that tablets promote good health. Since this worker believes in the benefit of iron tablets, she takes this opinion as fact and does not check further before adding these tablets as a supplement to her patient's diet. The problem is that, in fact, these iron tablets are not necessary for everyone's diet and may even be harmful if the patient has an allergic reaction to the tablets. A health care worker cannot administer tablets based on an opinion expressed in an article. Administration of supplements to diets must be based on physician's orders and on the facts stated on the patient's chart. Your opinion as a health care worker is not a valid basis for adding supplements to a patient's diet.

Example 2–4

Suppose you were asked to demonstrate to your supervisor that safety conditions in your work environment need to be improved. You would first have to establish as a fact that the safety conditions do need to be upgraded.

For example, if your task were to prepare a report on improving the fire drills in your health care institution, you would first prepare a checklist of procedures to follow during a fire drill. These procedures are the facts you would apply to measure the effectiveness of fire drills in your work or school environment.

Read the following selection on fire drills from *Saunders Fundamentals for Nursing Students* (Polaski and Warner, pp. 303-304). Seven procedures are listed for fire drills. These procedures, or facts, will help you to decide if your institution needs to improve its fire drill instructions.

Fire Drills

Every health care institution holds unannounced fire drills on all shifts so employees can practice the steps to take in case of fire. Team work is important. Each health care institution expects its staff to respond to a fire drill. You need to know what actions are expected of you during a drill. Until the all-clear signals sound after a fire drill, you should act as though a real fire is burning in the institution.

If you ever spot a fire, you should immediately do the following:

1. Sound the nearest fire alarm.
2. Notify the appropriate person of the fire's location.
3. Assist patients to a safe place away from the fire by using stairways. *Never* use the elevator during a fire.
4. Use a fire extinguisher when the fire is small and nearby on the unit.
5. Turn off electrical equipment in the area of the fire (if it is safe to do so).
6. Turn off any oxygen in use (if it is safe to do so).
7. Close doors and windows.

Directions: Use the seven facts above to evaluate the fire drill procedures in your work or school environment. Do these facts support the opinion that your institution needs to improve its fire drill safety procedures? Why? Why not?

Write a report evaluating the fire drill procedures in your school or workplace. Base your evaluation on the seven facts you have read in this selection.

_____

_____

_____

_____

_____

_____

_____

_____

_____

_____

_____

_____

_____

_____

_____

_____

▼ EVALUATING DIFFERENTIATING FACT FROM OPINION

Sometimes you have to form an opinion based on facts that you are given. Your action will be based on the judgment you have formed. Therefore it is important that you have all the facts possible and that your facts are accurate before you form an opinion.

A health care worker notices an open bottle of pills in a hospital room. The patient cannot be aroused. The health care worker has to examine the three obvious facts.

1. The bottle of sleeping pills is open.
2. Half the pills are missing.
3. The patient cannot be aroused.

Therefore the health care worker can form a judgment that this patient swallowed too many pills and help is needed immediately. The three facts make this decision a valid judgment.

Example 2–5

Read this evaluation from *Saunders Fundamentals for Nursing Assistants* (Polaski and Warner, p. 277). Notice that the phrase "undesirable behavior" is underlined. This opinion or judgment that the behaviors are "undesirable" is justified by the facts given.

Safety in Young and Middle-Aged Adults

From the early 20s through the 60s (as well as older adults), the person who is a patient in the health care institution may be exposed to danger as a result of smoking, drinking alcohol, or abusing drugs. These are all considered substance abuse. Be alert to signs of <u>undesirable behaviors</u> such as the following:

- the smell of cigarette or cigar smoke in the room
- the presence of matches in the wastebasket
- lighters on the bedside stand
- the presence of medications from home
- unusual behavior
- inappropriate answers to simple questions

Directions: Read the following selection from *Saunders Fundamentals for Nursing Assistants* (Polaski and Warner, p. 281). Examine the facts given. Based on the facts given, write your opinion: Do you think a health care institution should permit smoking? Why? Why not?

Smoking

The nurse will give you special instructions on how to handle patients who smoke cigarettes or cigars. The patients who are sedated are not permitted to smoke unless a care giver is present. If patients are confused or wandering, you may be asked to remain with them while they smoke. You should perform the following safety measures in this case:

- Provide a proper container for the disposal of ashes while patients smoke
- Do not discard cigarette or cigar butts or ashes into plastic waste containers.
- Place the burning end into a container of sand to extinguish the fire.
- Store matches, lighters, cigarettes, and cigars in a safe place.

Some health care institutions desire a smoke-free environment and do not allow any smoking on the premises. Other institutions may permit smoking in designated areas of the building. Always follow the nurse's direction regarding patients or visitors who smoke.

_____

_____

CRITICAL READING

Previewing

Preview this selection. Think about what you already know concerning this topic. In the space provided, write what you still wish to know.

_____

_____

_____

_____

_____

_____

_____

Questioning

Based on your preview, formulate questions that will help you learn what you still wish to know about the topic. Use the space provided.

_____

_____

_____

_____

_____

Reading

Read the following selection from *EMT Prehospital Care* (Henry and Stapleton, pp. 736-738).

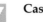

Case History

You respond to an automobile accident in which there are injured occupants. The questions that should go through your mind as you approach the scene include the following: How many casualties will there be? How did the accident occur? Will assistance be needed? Is the victim trapped? Upon your arrival, you find two vehicles. One victim is pinned by the steering wheel in vehicle number one and two victims are in vehicle number two. The arm of the driver of vehicle number two is trapped in the space between his seat and the door post, and his feet are caught beneath the pedals. The head of the passenger in vehicle number two has been thrust through the windshield and is stuck. These situations present problems that have relatively simple solutions. However, unless you learn the skills of extrication and how to apply them, this scenario could result in unnecessary tragedy.

Rescue of the entrapped victim is a specialized field. However, it is important for the EMT to be familiar with the use of basic hand tools and the principles of extrication.

Introduction

Freeing the trapped accident victim represents a challenging aspect of prehospital care. The stressful combination of a confined working environment; the trapped, unstable patient; and the surrounding chaos tests the nerves and stamina of the EMT. Early after your arrival you should determine whether additional resources are needed to attend to the multiple tasks required to save the victims. Fortunately, many EMS systems provide a separate division of rescue personnel to support the EMT in his or her extrication efforts.

Role of the EMT

At the accident scene, the EMT's primary role is evaluation and emergency care. Proper assessment and treatment along with careful packaging of the patient for removal should be foremost in your mind. However, if rescue crews are not available, you should be sufficiently confident to carry out an efficient and safe extrication.

The availability of specialized crews for rescue varies from one locale to another. In cities, there are often separate rescue teams who specialize in extrication and rescue. EMTs must know how to rapidly access this needed support. The EMT in such an area does not have to maintain as high a degree of proficiency in rescue operations as does an EMT located in a place where such support does not exist. EMTs in rural or suburban areas may be required to be more proficient in extrication skills. In some locales, the EMTs may also function as the specialists in rescue and extrication—skills obtained from training beyond the EMT curriculum.

Regardless of where you work, it is desirable for all EMTs to have a basic knowledge of extrication and be proficient in the use of light extrication tools. The EMT's ability to make the distinction between light and heavy rescue circumstances is critical.

A light rescue situation is one in which an extrication can be accomplished through the use of hand tools and basic skills such as sliding the seat back, applying a short spine board, and removing the patient. A heavy rescue situation is one in which power tools and additional resources and personnel are required. The EMT must be able to quickly determine if light or heavy rescue services are needed as well as to assess if he or she is capable of handling the situation.

If rescue personnel are available, your role is to ensure proper assessment, treatment, and removal of the patient. EMTs should coordinate their efforts with rescue personnel.

Scene Safety

One of the most basic principles of rescue operations is that the scene must be assessed for potential danger to rescuers, the public, and the patient. It is important to recognize that not all patients who are in need of rescue can be rescued. There are certain situations that present such significant hazards to both rescuers and the public that an effort to effect the rescue may be both futile and costly (in terms of lives). The need to do a risk-benefit analysis is essential. The rescuer who runs into a burning building without assessing the safety of the scene and loses his or her life becomes an additional victim unnecessarily.

A classic example of a failure to assess hazards occurred several years ago. An EMT crew responding to a report of a child who had fallen into a pit entered a toxic environment without regard for their personal safety. They also failed to don their protective clothing and breathing apparatus. It is very difficult to critique the actions of individuals who have given their lives in an effort to effect a rescue; however, it is important to analyze and learn from past mistakes to prevent future loss of life.

In the case mentioned above, when the ambulance arrived, a father stated that his child had fallen into a pit that was used to store grass clippings. The EMTs entered this environment without the benefit of self-contained breathing apparatus. The first EMT entered the pit and found the child but was overcome by toxic fumes. The second EMT, seeing his partner in need of help, tried to rescue him and was overcome as well. Upon the arrival of the volunteer fire department, one of the firefighters who knew the EMTs also entered the pit without benefit of a self-contained breathing apparatus. This individual also succumbed to the toxic fumes. The child for whom the original rescue had been initiated was subsequently retrieved and resuscitated. The lives of the three individuals who attempted the rescue were lost.

Your protective "envelope" represents the single most important factor in reducing EMT injury. A complete protective envelope consists of headgear, eye protection, respiratory protection (if required), gloves, boots, and coat. In dealing with a rescue situation, it is essential to remember that patient care always precedes the rescue effort *unless a life safety hazard exists*. A life safety hazard is any situation in which the rescuers are risking serious injury or death as the result of entering the rescue area. A life safety hazard is encountered, for example, every time an EMT stops to assist an injured motorist on a dark, unmarked roadway. Remember, your value to the patient is lost if you are injured or killed.

The greatest and most common hazard encountered by EMTs is the traffic surrounding auto accidents. The wearing of dark clothing, the failure to don reflective vests, and the inappropriate use of traffic delineation devices, all present unnecessary risks to EMTs. Traffic cones, flares, and the lights on the ambulance should be used to alert oncoming traffic that there is a hazard ahead and to protect those operating at the scene. While traffic control is usually a police function, situations occur that require EMTs to be knowledgeable about traffic hazards. Many EMTs have been badly injured and killed in traffic situations. The EMT must be alert to traffic hazards at all times.

Once the hazards are eliminated and you are wearing your protective clothing, the medical treatment for the entrapped patient becomes your priority. In this type of operation, your rapid assessment and treatment abilities are put to the test. The need for an accurate, focused approach is paramount because of the distractions of the environment.

Since most auto accidents involve more than one patient, it is important that the EMTs involved in the rescue effort perform triage prior to treatment. The ability to skillfully triage patients in an auto extrication situation may be hampered by limited access to the trapped victims. Additionally, the extrication time necessary to remove a patient may change the triage status of the patient. For instance, a patient who is a yellow priority (e.g., an individual with long bone fractures who is experiencing significant internal bleeding) might have to be recategorized as a red if the estimated extrication time is prolonged.

Time on the Scene

Since the trauma patient often requires surgical intervention in order to stabilize his or her condition, time is an important consideration in every rescue. As soon as possible, the patient must be evaluated to determine the need for lifesaving management, including rapid transport to a trauma center. The concept of time must be foremost in the mind of the rescuer, especially when several victims are entrapped and priorities must be established.

Patient care should include attention to life-threatening injuries; immobilization; and, when possible, rapid extrication. All patients should be immobilized to prevent further injury during the rescue effort.

Applying

In the space provided, answer your questions.

_____

_____

_____

_____

_____

_____

_____

_____

_____

_____

_____

Evaluating

Were you able to answer all your questions? Yes _____ No _____ . Did the selection give you enough information about the topic? Explain.

_____

_____

_____

_____

_____

_____

_____

_____

_____

_____

_____

Check the accuracy of your answers by finding the specific information in the selection.

STUDENT JOURNAL

List what you have learned about differentiating fact from opinion.	How would you apply this knowledge to your study or work in the health fields?

Chapter 3

Detecting Biases

EXERCISE
3-1

▼ **LEARNING OBJECTIVES**

In this chapter you will learn how to

- Detect biases in your readings, personal life, and workplace.

▼ **PREDICTING VOCABULARY**

Directions: Preview this chapter by finding five words that you recognize but whose precise definition you don't know. Use your background knowledge to write a sentence for each word that predicts the definition of that word.

Word 1: _____

Sentence: _____

_____

Word 2: _____

Sentence: _____

_____

Word 3: _____

Sentence: _____

_____

Word 4: _____

Sentence: _____

_____

Word 5: _____

Sentence: _____

_____

When you finish reading this chapter, evaluate the accuracy of your sentences. Make any necessary revisions.

Revisions

_____

_____

_____

_____

_____

_____

_____

_____

_____

_____

▼ UNDERSTANDING DETECTING BIASES

Biases are the prejudices or feelings you have about people, ideas, or circumstances. In some instances these biases are positive or admirable. For example, you may favor 18-year-olds' going on for further education after high school rather than hanging around the neighborhood. You can then say that you are biased toward more schooling for young people. In other instances biases can be negative or harmful. For example, as an employer, you refuse to hire anyone who appears to be over 50 years old to work in the hospital. Consequently, you can be described as someone who is biased against older people. Biases, then, are the leanings and notions you may have for or against certain groups, ideas, or experiences. We all have biases. However, as a health care student, you have the responsibility to recognize biases in the material you read so that you will have greater critical understanding of the texts. Similarly, you have the responsibility to recognize biases in your thinking so that you will improve your performance in the workplace.

One way writers show their biases is by their choice of words. Many words have two types of meanings, **denotation** and **connotation.** Denotation refers to the dictionary-type meaning of a word. For instance, "skinny" means "thin." But the word "skinny" suggests something else. It is usually used in an unflattering way to describe someone thin. This unflattering suggestion implied in the word "skinny" is the connotation of the word. The connotation usually has an emotional meaning attached to it. Because of this emotional association, words can indicate the writer's biases. A writer who uses "slim" to describe thinness feels more favorable toward thinness than a writer who uses "gaunt." Recognizing the positive and negative connotations of words is a great first step in detecting biases in readings.

Directions: Below are pairs of words. Read each word or short phrase and label it "N" if the word or phrase has a negative connotation or "P" if the word or phrase has a positive connotation.

1. assertive _____   aggressive _____
2. curious _____   nosy _____
3. crippled _____   physically challenged _____
4. full-figured _____   fat _____
5. reserved _____   withdrawn _____
6. stubborn _____   determined _____
7. young _____   immature _____
8. zealous _____   earnest _____
9. smell _____   aroma _____
10. thrifty _____   cheap _____

Directions: Using the space provided and in your own words, discuss what connotation and denotation mean. Give examples to support your ideas.

_____

_____

_____

_____

_____

_____

_____

_____

_____

_____

_____

_____

_____

_____

_____

_____

▼ INTERPRETING DETECTING BIASES

Now that you recognize that word choice might indicate the writer's bias, you are ready to look at the larger picture—detecting bias in reading passages. It is important to keep in mind that when writers write, they are expressing their belief or attitude on a topic. When writers take a position, they are advancing one outlook over another. This is bias. As a critical reader, you need to determine when a writer is presenting a biased report on a subject. To accomplish this, you should follow these strategies:

1. Know enough about the subject. You must have sufficient **background knowledge** of the topic to recognize any bias.
2. Understand the writer's arguments. Your vocabulary and reading **comprehension** must be good enough to grasp the writer's outlook. You can then begin to identify any bias.
3. Be aware of your **personal biases** on the topic. To fully understand the writer's position and bias, you must be able to sort them out from your own. Then you will be able to interpret the passage more accurately and detect any of the writer's bias.

Example 3–1

Below is a quotation from *The Medical Assistant: Administrative and Clinical* (Kinn, Woods, and Derge, p. 689). Following the quotation is an explanation of how one reader used the preceding strategies to identify the writer's bias.

According to Marion Nestle, professor of nutrition at New York University and an advisor to government nutrition agencies:

> The standard four food groups are based on American agriculture lobbies. Why do we have a milk group? Because we have a national dairy council. Why do we have a meat group? Because we have an extremely powerful meat lobby.

Strategy 1: Background Knowledge

I remember studying about the four food groups when I was in sixth grade. The four food groups were meat, grains, vegetables and fruits, and dairy. We were told how much of these foods we needed to eat daily to stay healthy.

Strategy 2: Comprehension

When I first read this quotation, I did not know what lobbies were. I looked it up in the dictionary and learned that lobbies are the different groups that try to influence lawmakers to pass certain laws. Also, I see that meat lobbies are described as "extremely powerful." In my mind this description connotes "unfair influence." I'm beginning to recognize some bias here.

Strategy 3: Personal Biases

Personally, I enjoy drinking milk and consider it a good source of calcium. I also don't mind a good steak occasionally. It seems reasonable to me that different interest groups would want to influence the government. That is a freedom we have in America. However, this writer seems to feel differently. The writer suggests that these lobbies are pressure groups looking out for their own interest. Even though our outlooks are different, I still believe that the writer was biased in this representation of agriculture's lobbying efforts.

Directions: Below is another excerpt from the Kinn, Woods, and Derge textbook (p. 689). Following the excerpt is a chart labeled with the three strategies for interpreting biases. After reading the passage carefully, try to determine if there is any bias in the passage by filling in how you thought through each of the three strategies. Refer to Example 3–1 if you need help.

Just before the "Eat Right Pyramid" was to be introduced to the American public, the Secretary of Agriculture unexpectedly suspended its release. Representatives from the dairy and meat industries, fearing negative economic repercussions, objected to the placement of their food groups next to the sweets and fats group near the top of the pyramid. The message was quite clear—governmental nutritional advice is driven as much by political and economic considerations as by scientific recommendations to improve public health; thus, each person has the responsibility to construct a healthy diet for himself or herself.

Strategy 1: Background Knowledge

_____

_____

_____

_____

Strategy 2: Comprehension

_____

_____

_____

_____

Strategy 3: Personal Biases

_____

_____

_____

_____

Directions: Based on the information in the excerpt in Exercise 3–4 and your own background knowledge, in the space provided write a different explanation for the secretary of agriculture's suspending the release of the Eat Right Pyramid. Be aware of the connotations of the key words in your explanation.

_____

_____

_____

_____

_____

_____

_____

_____

_____

_____

_____

_____

▼ APPLYING DETECTING BIASES

As a thoughtful person, you probably have many feelings on an array of subjects. Some of these feelings are positive, while others may be negative. This is natural. However, when you become a health care worker, it will be your responsibility in the workplace not to act on the negative feelings or prejudices you may have. To do so would be considered discrimination. You must try to detect your own biases and act fairly toward all. For example,

Lyndsay F., a dental assistant, was aware of her biases toward people who received public assistance. Since Lyndsay worked in a large dental clinic, many of the people being served fell into this category. However, instead of giving in to her prejudices and being miserable on the job, Lyndsay decided that it was in her own best interest to put this negative bias aside. She tried viewing patients who received public assistance as individuals with needs rather than grouping them or stereotyping them as welfare sorts. Lyndsay solved her bias problem by being more empathetic, or understanding, of others' circumstances. In addition, Lyndsay discussed her efforts to overcome her biases with her co-workers, many of whom shared her prejudices. This open discussion helped the others work through their own negative feelings, and eventually the working conditions and morale at the clinic improved for employees and patients alike.

Directions: Following are workplace situations that may involve bias. In the space provided, write how you would solve each of the problems.

Problem 1: An overweight person comes to you applying for a position as a front desk receptionist in the ophthalmologist's office.

_____

_____

_____

_____

_____

Problem 2: As a phlebotomist, you suspect that you are taking blood from a number of gay individuals.

_____

_____

_____

_____

_____

Problem 3: You are a religious person working in an obstetrics clinic that is responsible for dispensing birth control items and education.

_____

_____

_____

_____

_____

Problem 4: You work for a psychiatrist who specializes in treating the marital problems of people with multiple divorces. You believe that marriages should last forever.

_____

_____

_____

_____

_____

Problem 5: Most of your fellow workers have more liberal outlooks and life-styles than you do.

_____

_____

_____

_____

_____

▼ EVALUATING DETECTING BIASES

Following is the code of conduct for medical technologists as endorsed by the American Society for Medical Technology:

Being fully cognizant of my responsibilities in the practice of Medical Technology, I affirm my willingness to discharge my duties with accuracy, thoughtfulness and care.

Realizing that the knowledge obtained concerning patients in the course of my work must be treated as confidential, I hold inviolate the confidences placed in me by patients and physicians.

Recognizing that my integrity and that of my profession must be pledged to the absolute reliability of my work, I will conduct myself at all times in a manner appropriate to the dignity of my profession. [Flynn, p. 7]

Ultimately your beliefs and actions, whether in your personal or work life, should be based on objective standards or codes created by your religion, family, community, or profession. As a health care student, you will be entering a field that holds principles like those stated in the Code of Conduct of the American Society of Medical Technology to be paramount. It is on this code of ethics or ones similar that you will begin to judge and evaluate whether what you are reading is biased or not. It is on this code of ethics or similar ones that you will judge and evaluate your own biases and actions in the workplace. And it is on this code of ethics or ones similar that you will judge and evaluate fellow workers' biases and actions. Learn your field's code of conduct and let it be your guide for detecting biases in your reading materials and working life.

Example 3–2

Derin, a medical transcriptionist, returned from vacation to discover a huge stack of tapes that needed to be transcribed. As she worked through the tapes, she came across one describing the condition of her best friend's partner who had contracted a sexually transmitted disease. Derin's first impulse was to call her friend and warn her about the partner's medical condition. However, Derin remembered reading the American Association For Medical Transcription Code of Ethics. One of the major points was concerned with protecting the privacy and confidentiality of medical records. Although Derin was inclined to warn her friend, her evaluation showed her that upholding the principles of her profession was more important. Derin acted against her personal bias but nonetheless felt she had chosen the proper action.

Directions: Below is an excerpt from *The Medical Assistnat: Administrative and Clinical* (Kinn, Woods, and Derge, p. 436) describing patient care for HIV (human immunodeficiency virus). Carefully read the excerpt and review the American Society for Medical Technology's Code of Conduct cited previously. In the space provided, indicate any examples of bias you found in either the choice of words or the content in the excerpt on patient care. Then write an evaluation of how well the suggestions given in the excerpt reflect the ideals stated in the Code of Conduct.

Caring for the HIV-Infected Patient

The patient who becomes chronically ill must cope with the emotional, physical, and psychologic aspects of his or her illness. When an individual is diagnosed with an HIV infection, the emotional reactions from family, friends, and health care workers are even more prevalent. These patients are often rejected and feared and are aware of such feelings among health care professionals. As a result, the HIV-infected patient often does not seek medical help. Medical assistants need to be aware of their own feelings before they can focus on the patient's needs.

All interactions with the HIV-infected patient should be based on honesty and fairness. The patient's needs and concerns should be the focal point. When a patient is coping with a life-threatening disease, making him or her feel socially isolated places an unwarranted psychologic burden.

Many HIV-infected patients may be either homosexual or bisexual, and prejudice toward them based on their lifestyle can have a negative impact on the manner in which they are treated. The medical assistant should not view the HIV-infected patient in a negative fashion. You may feel that this patient deserves the illness and deserves to die, but these feelings must remain personal and not be reflected in the quality of the care given.

As health care workers, we must remember that the HIV-infected person has a legal right to total health care. Every patient needs to be given comfort and compassion when afflicted with chronic and possibly terminal illnesses. The medical assistant can be the patient's advocate and an aid to the physician by showing genuine concern for the welfare of the HIV-infected patient and by gaining the trust and the cooperation of the patient.

For more than a century, it has been a recognized fact that infections and infectious body specimens pose an occupational hazard to the health care worker, but never has any disease posed a more serious threat than AIDS. Fear and hysteria are commonplace, and many competent health care workers have left the profession as a result.

Every paper, magazine, and professional journal that you read has at least one article on HIV or AIDS. Many of these articles contradict each other, leaving the reader to wonder what the truth is and who can be believed.

The medical assistant *must* learn to follow the universal precautions and not attempt a "short cut" in order to complete a task more quickly. Integrity and honesty must be the prime virtues in coping with this disease and with the patients who have it. It is only through education that this disease can be brought under control, and only when it is under control can the health care worker claim victory.

AIDS is a very sensitive subject for all of us, but it may not disappear for a long time to come. In the very near future, every medical practice will include an HIV-positive patient. If you have a problem working with AIDS and HIV-infected patients, it may be wise for you to reconsider your vocational goal of working in the medical field.

Examples of Bias

_____

_____

_____

_____

_____

_____

_____

Evaluation of Suggestions

_____

_____

_____

_____

_____

_____

_____

_____

CRITICAL READING

Previewing

Preview this selection. Think about what you already know concerning this topic. In the space provided, write what you still wish to know.

_____

_____

_____

_____

_____

Questioning

Based on your preview, formulate questions that will help you learn what you still wish to know about the topic. Use the space provided.

Reading

Read the following selection from *Procedures in Phlebotomy* (Flynn, pp. 189-193):

Other Legal Doctrines and Areas of Law Applicable to Phlebotomy Practice

Interplay Among the Rights of Privacy, Confidentiality, and Informed Consent

The issues litigated in legal disputes involving intentional and unintentional injury to patients and clients by health care workers have their roots in guaranteed individual rights. These rights have their basis in the United States Constitution and Bill of Rights, regardless of whether they are specifically enumerated in the Constitution. For example, the U.S. Constitution does not mention a right of privacy; however, the United States Supreme Court has recognized that a right of privacy exists and that certain areas of privacy are guaranteed under the Constitution. The right of privacy includes the right to confidentiality, and if this right is waived, consent to the waiver must be informed.

Right of Privacy. An individual's right "to be let alone," recognized in all United States jurisdictions, includes the right to be free of "intrusion upon physical and mental solitude or seclusion" and the right to be free of "public disclosure of private facts." Every health care institution and health care worker has a duty to respect a patient's or client's right of privacy, which includes the privacy and confidentiality of information obtained from the patient/client for purposes of diagnosis, medical records, and public health reporting requirements. If a health care worker conducts tests on or publishes information about a patient/client without that person's consent, the health care worker could be sued for wrongful invasion of privacy, **defamation,** or a variety of other actionable torts.

Confidentiality. Health care workers must be vigilant in keeping information about patients and clients confidential. This is especially true in blood banks, transfusion services, and phlebotomy services, where phlebotomists may have access to information about patients who are human immunodeficiency virus (HIV)–positive, have acquired immunodeficiency syndrome (AIDS) or other sexually transmitted diseases, or who may have medical histories that, if disclosed, might cause undue embarrassment to or prejudice or discrimination against that patient. Phlebotomists and their supervisors should understand that they have a legal duty to keep records, documentation, and laboratory test results confidential. This duty may be waived only if a patient has given express permission for the information to be released, if the patient has sued the institution or its health care personnel, or if the health care worker is specifically obligated to release patient information (e.g., to the Centers for Disease Control and Prevention or other authorized public health department). Even in the last situation, care must be taken to ensure that the confidentiality of patient records and reports cannot be breached while they are being communicated or are in transit.

Consent and Informed Consent. Physicians and other health care workers are required to obtain a patient's consent before performing any invasive or diagnostic procedure. Consent can take a variety of forms (e.g., written agreements, spoken words, implicit actions, or making an appointment for a test). In a nineteenth century case, for example, a plaintiff's failure to object to a vaccine that the defendant was preparing to give to the plaintiff conveyed apparent consent to the injection.

However, to agree to a medical procedure, a patient must first know what he or she is agreeing to. Thus, the doctrine of consent has expanded to include *informed consent,* which emphasizes that health care workers must fully disclose any risks, alternatives, and benefits of a procedure or test so that the patient/client can make an informed decision about whether he or she wants to be treated or tested. "[T]he doctrine of informed consent imposes on a physician, before he subjects his patient to medical treatment, the duty to explain the procedure to the patient and to warn him of any material risks or dangers inherent in or collateral to the therapy, so as to enable the patient to make an intelligent and informed choice about whether or not to undergo such treatment."

The correlate to informed consent is *informed refusal.* Patients may refuse treatment for religious, social, financial, or other reasons, but even in these cases a health care worker may be found negligent for the lack of information given to the patient, if the patient didn't have enough information available to make a reasonable decision to forego treatment.

In general, it is the physician who has the duty to disclose adequate information to a patient. Phlebotomists should be wary of volunteering information to a patient in situations where they do not have the legal or professional authority to do so. These situations may be difficult "judgment calls" for the phlebotomist, as patients often ask phlebotomists questions about their treatment or why they are drawing blood. The phlebotomist should politely refer the patient to his or her physician or charge nurse for these explanations.

Patient's Bill of Rights

In the early 1970s, the American Hospital Association developed a policy statement for health care institutions and their patients that incorporated and reflected the individual rights guaranteed under the legal doctrines of privacy, informed consent, and confidentiality. Since that time, many hospitals have adopted the *Patient's Bill of Rights* into their policy manuals, and some state legislatures have passed Patient's Bill of Rights statutes.

The *Patient's Bill of Rights* is intended to "promote the interests and well-being of the patients and residents of health care facilities." As such, it enumerates the patient's right to respectful care, to adequate information with which to make an informed decision (or refusal) about his or her care, and to confidentiality in treatment and communication of records about his or her medical care program. In addition, the document affirms a patient's right to information about medical bills and charges, possible involvement in medical research and experimentation, and hospital rules and regulations.

Medical Devices and Equipment Failures

Phlebotomists use many pieces of equipment or reagents that are manufactured by medical equipment or pharmaceutical companies and then purchased by the hospital or laboratory from manufacturers, distributors, or retailers. These supplies—whether they be needles, syringes, protective equipment or clothing, chemicals, or blood—may, in unusual situations, be defective or unsafe because of the way they were designed, assembled, or screened, or they may be inherently dangerous even when used under normal conditions. When a patient suffers a needle break during blood drawing, has a violent reaction to a drug, or contracts an infectious disease after use of a product, he or she may sue the manufacturer of that product under various legal theories, including negligence, strict liability in tort, and breach of *implied warranty of merchantability*.

Under negligible theory, plaintiffs must prove that defendants have a duty to conform to certain standards of care in the manufacture of their products and to guard against unreasonable risks. *Strict liability in tort* is imposed when manufacturers are held liable for injuries caused by an unreasonably dangerous or defective product, even if there is no finding of fault. Breach of an implied warranty of merchantability may be found, on the basis that manufacturers or sellers of goods should be obligated to provide consumers with products that are fit for the purpose for which they are being sold.

These legal actions fall under the law of *products liability*. Products liability focuses on the liability of suppliers for defective products that cause physical harm. The defect in question may not be the actual product itself; defects may arise because of inadequate packaging, instructions, or warning labels.

The term "product" implies goods that are sold predominantly in commercial settings. Manufacturer liability for defective health care products has received much professional and legal attention, because health care treatment and diagnostic testing has traditionally been viewed as a service rather that as a product. Especially in the areas of blood transfusions (which may result in HIV transmission) and genetically engineered pharmaceuticals (such as coagulation components), the distinction between products and services has been challenged by plaintiffs who sue blood banks or pharmaceutical companies to recover damages resulting from transmission of infectious diseases.

Because the availability of blood and blood products is of great importance to public health, many states have passed blood shield statutes that exempt blood transfers, blood derivatives, or blood products from the threat of products liability lawsuits and specifically mandate that blood components are to be considered medical services, not goods or products. **Immunity** from legal action thus guarantees an adequate blood supply for use in medical emergencies and treatment of chronic blood-related disorders.

Case Law

As the range of health care services has expanded and health care personnel have become more specialized, the reach of malpractice **litigation** is no longer confined to the physician-patient relationship and may include nonmedical personnel as part of the health care team. Although most of the following cases did not specifically involve phlebotomists, the situations in which these claims arose can be readily analogized to laboratory and phlebotomy practice. These cases do not represent an exhaustive review of phlebotomy-related malpractice but are intended to remind phlebotomists of problems that may develop when practice standards and procedures are compromised.

Belmon v St. Frances Cabrini Hospital, 427 So2d 541, 544 (LaApp, 1983) [Negligent blood sample collection by a medical technician caused hemorrhage.]

Butler v Louisiana State Board of Education, 331 So2d 192, 196 (LaApp, 1976) [A donor fainted and sustained injuries, and a biology professor was held negligent for not giving students previous instructions on blood drawing and donor care.]

St. Paul Fire and Marine Insurance Co v Prothro, 590 SW2d 35 (Ark App 1979) [Negligent physical therapy procedures caused a patient to develop a *Staphylococcus* infection.]

Simpson v Sisters of Charity of Providence, 588 P2d 4 (Or 1978) [Radiology technician performed a poor-quality radiograph that failed to demonstrate a fracture that subsequently caused paralysis.]

Southeastern Kentucky Baptist Hospital, Inc v Bruce, 539 SW2d 286 (Ky 1976) [Misidentification of a patient led to a surgical procedure on the wrong patient.]

Wood v Miller, 76 P2d 963 (Or 1983) [Negligent use of diathermy equipment burned a patient.]

Favalora v Aetna Casualty and Surety Co, 144 So2d 544 (La App 1962) [A patient fainted and fell, causing injuries; a radiology technician and supervising physician were found negligent for not being alert to and prepared for the patient's condition.]

McCormick v Auret (Ga 1980) [Failure to use sterile equipment during venipuncture led to nerve damage secondary to infection.]

Alessio v Crook, 633 SW2d 770 (Tenn App 1982) [Failure to include an x-ray report in the patient's medical record before patient discharge resulted in more extensive surgery than would have been required had the physician seen the report.]

Variety Children's Hospital v Osle, 292 So2d 382 (Fl App D3 1974) [A surgeon failed to label and separate specimens sent to a pathology laboratory. Because the pathologist was unable to determine which of the two specimens was malignant, removal of both of the patient's breasts was necessary.]

Jeanes v Milner, 428 F2d 598 (Ark 1970) [A 1-month delay in mailing specimens to a laboratory resulted in delayed diagnosis of cancer; if it had been detected promptly and treated, the pain and suffering of the patient could have been lessened.]

Ray v Wagner, 176 NW2d 101 (Minn 1970) [A patient claimed a physician was negligent for failing to timely notify her of her malignancy; the patient was found contributorily negligent for giving the physician incomplete and misleading information about how she could be reached.]

Thor v Boska, 113 Cal Rptr 296 (1974) [A physician's inability to produce medical records after he had been sued for malpractice created an inference of guilt.]

Lauro v Travelers Insurance Company, 262 So2d 787 (La App 1972) [A hospital was not negligent for not using the latest laboratory equipment available, where current standards of care demonstrated that the equipment used was acceptable.]

Applying

In the space provided, answer your questions.

_____

_____

_____

_____

_____

_____

_____

Evaluating

Were you able to answer all your questions? Yes _____ No _____
Did the selection give you enough information about the topic? Explain.

_____

_____

_____

_____

_____

_____

Check the accuracy of your answers by locating the specific information in the selection.

STUDENT JOURNAL

List what you have learned about detecting biases.	How would you apply this knowledge to your study or work in the health fields?

Chapter 4

Making Value Judgments

▼ LEARNING OBJECTIVES

In this chapter you learn how to
- Make value judgments based on facts
- Avoid allowing emotionally charged words to influence your ability to make value judgments

▼ PREDICTING VOCABULARY

Directions: Preview this chapter by finding five words that you recognize but whose precise definition you don't know. Use your background knowledge to write a sentence for each word that predicts the definition of that word.

EXERCISE 4-1

Word 1: _____

Sentence: _____

_____

Word 2: _____

Sentence: _____

_____

Word 3: _____

Sentence: _____

_____

Word 4: _____

Sentence: _____

_____

Word 5: _____

Sentence: _____

_____

When you finish reading this chapter, evaluate the accuracy of your sentences. Make any necessary revisions.

Revisions

_____

_____

_____

_____

_____

_____

_____

_____

▼ UNDERSTANDING MAKING VALUE JUDGMENTS FROM READINGS

Making value judgments is one of your most difficult challenges as a critical reader and thinker. You must be an active reader and weigh the evidence presented before you make any judgments. As you read, you should avoid allowing emotionally charged words to influence your ability to make value judgments. Many writers deliberately choose words to create an emotional impact. If you react emotionally, it may cloud your thinking and prevent you from evaluating the information objectively.

Example 4–1

The following three sentences describe similar situations. Read them carefully and think about the emotional impact made by the italicized words.

1. The technician read the x-ray.
2. The technician _grimly studied_ the x-ray.
3. The technician _quickly glanced_ at the x-ray.

These examples show how even one or two words can alter the reader's emotional reaction to a sentence. Sentence 1 is objective; there is no emotional reaction on the part of the reader. Sentence 2 has a negative emotional impact. The words _grimly_ and _studied_ make the reader feel that something might be wrong with the results shown in the x-ray. Sentence 3 gives the reader the feeling that there was nothing to worry about. The words _quickly_ and _glanced_ convey a casual feeling.

As a critical reader and thinker, practice looking for emotionally charged words and avoid allowing these words to affect your ability to make value judgments.

Directions: Read the following sentences. Write whether each sentence is objective, positive, or negative. In each sentence, underline the words that create a positive or negative impact.

_____ 1. The emergency technicians raced to treat the victims of the devastating accident.

_____ 2. The nursing assistant took the patient's temperature.

_____ 3. The nursing assistant monitored the patient's rising temperature.

_____ 4. The nurse dispensed the patient's medication.

_____ 5. The nurse tried to lessen the patient's discomfort with prescribed painkillers.

_____ 6. The patient took a seat in the clinic.

_____ 7. The patient was relieved to find a vacant seat in the busy clinic.

_____ 8. Lisa's new contact lenses were comfortable, as well as flattering to her appearance.

_____ 9. The nutritionist prescribed a diet for the patient.

_____ 10. The obese patient was ordered to lose 80 pounds.

Once you have learned to recognize words that have an emotional impact, you will be careful to look for these emotionally charged words and not allow them to sway your thinking.

Directions: Examine the information in the following passage. Pay attention to the underlined words, which are emotionally charged. Then answer the questions.

Margorie wanted to lose 25 pounds. One of her friends took her to a diet counselor who promised startling results with a fad diet. When Margorie asked about the nutritional value of the diet, she was told to leave that worry to the experts. When she asked how long it should take her to lose 25 pounds, the counselor assured her that the weight would be off in no time. Margorie paid the fee and joined this weight loss program. Although she lost a few pounds at first, she started feeling weak and dizzy. She wasn't able to continue with the diet and felt like a failure for dropping out of the weight loss program.

1. What words or phrases were used to give Margorie a positive feeling about the weight loss program? _____

_____

2. How did these emotionally charged words affect Margorie's ability to make a value judgment? _____

_____

3. What facts should Margorie have had before she joined the weight loss program? _____

_____

Directions: Read the following selection from *Saunders Fundamentals for Nursing Assistants* (Polaski and Warner, p. 535).

Dietary guidelines issued by the U.S. Department of Agriculture help individuals meet their needs for nutrition. These guidelines suggest that individuals

- Eat a variety of foods.
- Maintain a desirable weight.
- Avoid too much fat and cholesterol.
- Eat food that has adequate starch and fiber.
- Avoid too much sugar.
- Avoid too much sodium (salt).
- Drink alcoholic beverages in moderation, if they are permitted.

Review Margorie's daily diet. Based on the dietary guidelines, decide whether this was a satisfactory weight loss program. Write those items from the dietary guidelines that helped you to make this judgment.

Breakfast	**Lunch**	**Dinner**
Orange juice	½ grapefruit	Salad
Banana	3 crackers/1 slice of toast	Tea, coffee, diet soda
	Tea or coffee (no sugar)	

_____

_____

▼ APPLYING MAKING VALUE JUDGMENTS FROM READINGS

Example 4-2

Margorie still had her weight problem. She needed to find a diet plan that would work for her. To make a value judgment, she had to examine the facts. She looked at the U.S. Department of Agriculture's list of five food groups.

The Five Food Groups

The U.S. Department of Agriculture has divided foods into five categories called food groups. The five food groups can be used to plan balanced meals. The five food groups are

- Fats, oils, and sweets
- Milk, yogurt, and cheese
- Meat, poultry, fish, dry beans, eggs, and nuts
- Vegetables and fruit
- Bread, cereal, rice, and pasta [Polaski and Warner, p. 528]

After Margorie examined this list, she made her own diet plan based on the five food groups:

Breakfast	Lunch	Dinner
Chocolate milkshake	Cheeseburger	Steak
Roll, butter	Fries	Rice
Cheese omelet	Soda	Salad
Orange juice	Apple pie	Chocolate cake
Coffee		Coffee

Although Margorie selected items from each food group, many of the selections on her daily diet were high-calorie, weight-increasing foods. Margorie clearly needed to get more information before she could make a value judgment in choosing a diet plan.

Directions: Carefully read Table 4–1 (p. 54), which gives information about the five food groups. Answer the following questions.

1. List three foods that are sources of protein.

   _____

   _____

   _____

2. If you were a vegetarian, what foods could you substitute for meat?

   _____

   _____

   _____

3. Which foods are sources of calcium?

   _____

   _____

   _____

4. Why should calcium be included in the daily diet? _____

   _____

Table 4–1 The Five Food Groups

Food Group	Examples	Benefits	Uses in the Body
Fats, oils, and sweets group	Cooking oils, lard, cake, candy bars	Fat	Helps body use fat-soluble vitamins
Milk, yogurt, and cheese group	Milk, cheese, ice cream, yogurt	Calcium	Tooth and bone growth
			Muscle function
		Protein	Muscle function
			Builds and repairs tissues
		Vitamins	Growth and health
Meat, fish, poultry, dry beans, eggs, and nuts group	Red meat (beef, pork), poultry (chicken, turkey)	Protein	Muscle function
			Builds and repairs tissue
		Vitamins	Growth and health
		Iron	Carries oxygen in the blood
Meat substitutes	Nuts, peanut butter, dry beans	Same as above	Same as above
Vegetable and fruit group	Green, leafy vegetables (lettuce, kale, and spinach); tomatoes; green beans; peas; corn; other vegetables; fruits such as apples, oranges, peaches, berries	Vitamins (mainly A and C)	Growth and health
Bread, cereal, rice, and pasta group	Breads: white, rye, wheat; cereals: bran, wheat, oat; pasta: macaroni, spaghetti, noodles	Vitamins Protein Iron	Growth and health Muscle function Carries oxygen in the blood

From Polaski A and Warner JP: Saunders fundamentals for nursing assistants, Philadelphia, 1994, WB Saunders, p. 528.

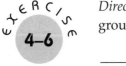

Directions: Using Table 4–1, plan a breakfast that would include all five groups.

_____

_____

_____

_____

_____

Margorie was becoming familiar with the five food groups. However, she needed help selecting low-calorie foods from the groups. She also decided to cut fat from her diet after reading the following information.

Directions: Read the following selection from *Saunders Fundamentals for Nursing Assistants* (Polaski and Warner, p. 527) and answer the questions that follow.

EXERCISE
4–7

Individuals should eat enough calories to produce the energy their body needs for tissue growth and repair and to get through the day. Complex carbohydrates (grain, cereal, fruit, and vegetables) provide the best energy bargain for the body. They give a person energy over a longer period of time because they take longer to digest and metabolize. Simple carbohydrates (donuts, potato chips, etc.) metabolize quickly and are easily stored as fat in the body. Protein (meat, dairy products) that is not used by the body may also be stored as fat. Fats (butter and oils) give the body energy when they are digested and metabolized, but they do not have much nutrient value. Any fat not used by the body is stored for reserve energy.

Example

If you eat 3 grams of carbohydrate, 4 grams of protein, and 2 grams of fat, which will give you the most calories?

3 grams carbohydrate = 12 calories

4 grams protein = 16 calories

2 grams fat = 18 calories

You might eat less fat, but it is high in calories.

1. Which foods provide the best energy bargain for the body?

   _____

2. Which foods are easily stored as fats?

   _____

Directions: Using Table 4–1 plan a low-calorie, low-fat breakfast. List the information in Table 4–1 and the reading in Exercise 4–7 that helped you to plan this breakfast.

EXERCISE
4–8

_____

_____

_____

_____

_____

_____

_____

_____

_____

▼ INTERPRETING MAKING VALUE JUDGMENTS

Margorie needed to find out more about food and health before she could select a diet plan so that she could make a value judgment on the best way for her to lose weight without sacrificing her health. Margorie read a selection on the essential nutrients from *Saunders Fundamentals for Nursing Assistants* (Polaski and Warner, p. 525) and learned, for example, that eliminating protein from her diet is a mistake because protein is necessary for cell growth and repair.

EXERCISE 4-9

Directions: Read the Polaski and Warner selection (p. 525) and answer the questions that follow based on the reading.

The essential nutrients needed for a healthy body have been identified by scientists. The nutrients are divided into the following groups.

Carbohydrates. Carbohydrates are a source of energy in the body and are found in sugar and starches. Carbohydrates that are not used are stored in the liver. When a person takes in too many carbohydrates, the excess sugar is changed into body fat and stored in the tissue. Simple carbohydrates, such as donuts or other bakery sweets, are those that the body uses quickly. A person may feel hungry soon after eating simple carbohydrates. Complex carbohydrates take longer for the body to break down and use. A person does not feel hunger as quickly when eating complex carbohydrates, such as cereals and grains. Cereals and grains include wheat, rice, oats, and bran. Fruits and vegetables are also sources of complex carbohydrates.

Protein. Protein is the material cells need to grow and to repair themselves. Protein is found in all body cells and all body fluids. In the diet, protein comes from meats, fish, poultry, eggs, milk, and dairy products.

Fat. Fat is another source of energy in the body. Another name for fat is adipose tissue. Fat is a concentrated form of energy that is stored in the body. Fats are important because they carry the fat-soluble vitamins (vitamins A, D, E, and K). Meats, dairy products such as milk and cheese, cooking oils, egg yolks, and nuts are rich sources of fat in the diet. Fat also includes cholesterol. **Cholesterol** is a fatty substance that attaches to the lining of arteries and makes them narrow. Too much cholesterol in your body can cause serious health problems.

Vitamins. **Vitamins** are essential elements needed in small amounts for a healthy body. Vitamins may be **fat-soluble** or **water-soluble.** The fat-soluble vitamins (A, D, E, and K) can be stored in the body's fat cells. Water-soluble vitamins cannot be stored and must be taken in by the body every day. Vitamin C and the B vitamins are water-soluble.

Minerals. **Minerals** are substances that work to help the body maintain good function. Minerals such as chloride, copper, phosphorus, fluoride, and many others are needed in various amounts. Minerals must be taken in by the body daily. They are important for good bones and teeth and help with nerve function. A varied diet that includes foods from the five food groups provides the amounts of vitamins and minerals needed for a healthy body. Minerals are found in almost all foods, except table sugar and oils.

Water. **Water** is a clear, odorless, tasteless fluid. Water carries important substances to the cell and takes away the waste products produced by the cell. Our bodies cannot survive for very long without water.

CHOLESTEROL
fatty substance that attaches to the lining of arteries; comes from animal fats and oils

VITAMIN
an organic substance that is essential in small amounts to the body's health

FAT-SOLUBLE
able to dissolve in fat

WATER-SOLUBLE
able to dissolve in water

MINERAL
an inorganic (neither animal nor vegetable) substance needed for health

WATER
clear, odorless, tasteless fluid

1. Which vitamins must be taken into the body every day? _____

_____

2. Why is drinking water important? _____

_____

3. Why are carbohydrates important to the body? _____

_____

4. How can too much cholesterol cause serious health problems? _____

_____

5. How can you be sure to include the amount of minerals and vitamins

needed for the body? _____

_____

Directions: Based on the reading in Exercise 4–9, choose which you would include in a breakfast menu, doughnuts or cereal. Explain why.

_____

_____

_____

_____

_____

▼ EVALUATING MAKING VALUE JUDGMENTS

Margorie now has to choose a diet plan based on the information she has read
and not be swayed by emotionally charged words. The following are examples of two diet plans Margorie examined:

Plan A

Breakfast	Lunch	Dinner
Cereal	Pasta, yogurt	Skinless chicken, fish, or turkey
Skim milk	Salad, vegetables	Salad
Fruit	Low-fat cottage cheese	Vegetables
Toast (one slice)	Tea or coffee	Baked potato
Tea or coffee		Tea or coffee
		Fruit
		Bread (one slice)

Plan B

Breakfast	Lunch	Dinner
Juice	Yogurt	Skinless chicken, fish, or turkey
Banana	Apple	Salad
Tea or coffee	Tea or coffee	Vegetable
		Diet soda
		Fruit
		Tea or coffee

Margorie chose plan A. She felt that she could not totally eliminate starch and carbohydrates from her diet. She also thought that plan B would leave her hungry, causing her to go off the diet.

Directions: Answer the following questions based on the preceding discussion.

1. Did she make a value judgment? Yes _____ No _____

2. Why? _____

_____

_____

Why not? _____

_____

_____

3. Which of the two diet plans would you choose for yourself?

   A _____   **B** _____

4. What information in this reading helped you to make this judgment?

_____

_____

_____

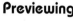

CRITICAL READING

Previewing

Think about what you already know about proper nutrition. In the space provided, write what you still wish to know.

_____

_____

_____

_____

_____

_____

Questioning

Based on your preview, formulate questions that will help you learn what you still wish to know about the topic.

_____

_____

_____

_____

_____

_____

Reading

Read the following selection from _EMT Prehospital Care_ (Henry and Stapleton, pp. 56-58).

The Patient History

The _history_ is frequently the most significant part of patient assessment. The history is the patient's story of significant events related to and surrounding the present problem that has necessitated seeking medical attention. The patient usually begins the history with words describing the main problem, which is called the _chief complaint_. This may be "Chest pain," "I can't breathe," or "It's the worst headache I've ever had." You should then go about a systematic and chronological gathering of relevant information associated with the chief complaint. This also includes pertinent past medical history.

Many serious diseases or conditions are often diagnosed primarily on the basis of history. For example, a heart attack victim is usually diagnosed in the prehospital setting based on information in his or her history.

The history is obtained by following a set sequence during the interview. This is done by all medical professionals to ensure collection of relevant data in an efficient manner. Properly taken, a history proceeds in an orderly fashion that allows information gathered to be processed together with physical signs to achieve a working diagnosis. Knowledge of signs and symptoms of diseases and injuries is essential. Throughout the following chapters, diseases and injuries are described by their clinical presentation.

The components of the history include *the chief complaint, the history of present illness, the past medical history, and medications and allergies.*

The history is the most subjective aspect of the diagnostic process. It relies upon the patient's description and interpretation rather than on objective findings directly observed, heard, or felt by the evaluator. Therefore, one should follow certain principles to maximize the validity and reliability of information gathered.

1. *Use open-ended questions.* As much as possible patients should express all complaints and facts in their own words. For example, if a patient complains of chest pain, the EMT should ask, "Can you describe the pain?" When the interviewer offers adjectives such as "Was this a sharp pain?" or "Did it feel like a burning sensation?" the interviewer runs the risk of "putting words in the patient's mouth." This would make the information far less reliable.

2. *Direct the interview.* Maintain the order of chief complaint, history of present illness, past medical history, and medications and allergies. This will ensure that relevant information is not overlooked. One component should lead to the next. Do not allow the patient to drift off the topic. Failure to maintain control can waste valuable time. Maintain the focus of the interview within relevant boundaries.

3. *Do not delay urgent treatments.* Although you should try to collect the most comprehensive history, it should not delay any therapy if an indication for such is evident. For example, oxygen therapy for a heart attack patient may be started as soon as the need has been determined. Other conditions may result in immediate transport. In any case, the history should be continued in the ambulance while en route to the hospital. This technique will achieve both important goals: RAPID INTERVENTION and MAXIMUM DATA COLLECTION.

4. *The patient is the best source for the history.* Keeping in mind that there are exceptions to this rule (an unconscious patient or small child), it is generally important to allow the patient to express the problem. Bystanders may interpret and misrepresent facts and, again, may put words in the patient's mouth. A bystander's history, while it may be important, should supplement rather than replace the patient's own history.

The direction that a history takes is very much determined by each developing fact. As you gain knowledge of signs, symptoms, and presentations of various disease states, this will become more evident to you. Like any investigative process, a single fact may alter your impression and your subsequent questioning. However, there are questions that are common to most complaints. These will be addressed as we discuss the various categories.

Chief Complaint. After learning basic facts about a patient (age and sex), you should ask the patient to describe the problem. The patient's single-sentence response becomes the chief complaint. Examples are "I woke up this morning with chest pain," "I have difficulty breathing," "I have a severe pain in my lower back." These statements will determine to some extent your follow-up questions.

If the patient's initial statement is too vague, such as "I feel sick," or "I hurt myself," you should request more specifics from the patient about the reason for calling for medical aid.

History of Present Illness. After the chief complaint is obtained, a series of questions are asked to expand and identify the cause of the chief complaint. The patient's activity at the time of the problem, a description of other associated symptoms, the sequence of events leading up to the incident, factors that aggravate or alleviate the problem, and similar past experiences are elicited at this time.

Throughout this text, these questions will be presented in the context of each critical condition. However, there are facts to be ascertained that are common to all complaints. The purpose of these questions is to identify the pattern of events that led up to, and is associated with, the immediate problem. These include:

1. *Sequence of events.* Have the patient express the order in which each sign or symptom occurred.

2. *Activity at the onset or immediately preceding the event.* Ask the patient to describe the activity involved when the problem first presented itself, e.g., running, sitting, walking up stairs, eating, and so forth.

3. *Aggravating and relieving factors.* Have the patient relate any behavior that makes the symptoms worse or alleviates them. For example, "Walking increases the pain" or "Sitting makes the pain go away."

4. *Similar past experiences.* Ask the patient if a similar problem has occurred before. If so, was a doctor consulted? Was there a hospital admission? What was the diagnosis? This line of questioning frequently identifies the cause.

5. *Associated symptoms.* Ask the patient if there are other complaints or abnormal sensations associated with the chief complaint. If there are no associated symptoms, you may ask about specific symptoms commonly associated with the chief complaint. For example, a person with severe abdominal pain who denies any associated symptoms might be questioned specifically about nausea and vomiting.

6. *Describing pain.* Questions about the complaint of "pain" should address several descriptive variables including location, duration, quality, severity, radiation (flow from one area to another), and aggravating and relieving factors.

During the *history of present illness,* you should start formulating a mental list of the possible causes of the patient's condition. The amount of information gathered during this phase will be determined by the effectiveness of your interview technique, as well as by the ability of the patient to respond. For example, brain hypoxia (poor oxygen delivery to the brain), drugs, disease states, and other factors may diminish thought processes and hamper the interview.

Past Medical History. One should always ask certain questions about a patient's past medical history for many reasons. It frequently clarifies or reinforces the diagnosis suspected from the history of the present illness. A variety of medical conditions are either progressive in nature (worsen over time) or are often associated with, or may aggravate, other conditions. A patient who has high blood pressure is at increased risk for a heart attack. Likewise, a history of *hemophilia* (a bleeding disorder) is of considerable importance when treating trauma patients.

When collecting the past medical history, the interviewer must use the time efficiently. Major illnesses requiring prior hospitalizations, illnesses presently under treatment, and illnesses similar to, or associated with, the present illness should be elicited. You may start this phase of the interview with open-ended questions such as "What major illnesses or injuries have you had in the past?" or "Are you undergoing treatment at this time?" This can be followed by more specific inquiries about diseases or injuries that may be related to the immediate condition.

In adult patients always inquire specifically about four conditions. These conditions can be remembered as "the big four" and include heart disease, hypertension (high blood pressure), diabetes, and chronic obstructive pulmonary disease (emphysema and bronchitis). These conditions can be progressive in nature, are risk factors for emergency conditions, and can alter treatment.

Medications and Allergies. Be sure to inquire specifically about an allergy history and whether the patient is taking any medications. Bring the medications to the hospital if they are readily available. An elderly person may not be able to describe the name of a specific disease that may be suspected by the need for a certain drug.

An allergy history may be useful for both prehospital diagnosis and as information to guide the choice of drug therapy in the hospital.

Medic Alert Tags. Some patients with a known disease such as diabetes or with severe allergies may wear or carry a Medic Alert tag or card. This bracelet, necklace, or wallet card may contain the only history available for an unconscious or disoriented patient. They may indicate specific conditions, medications, allergies, or other personal information needed to institute care.

Confidentiality

Information given to a medical practitioner is confidential and privileged information. You are entrusted to keep confidential both personal and medical information elicited during your patient interviews. Whenever possible, care should be taken to conduct the interview in a private setting. For example, in the workplace you should clear bystanders and co-workers from the immediate area before asking medical questions. While this may be modified by the patient's condition and the surroundings, it should still be a fundamental rule of practice. Conduct the interview with the same respect you would want shown to yourself or your family.

Summary

Becoming a skillful interviewer requires adherence to the structure outlined above and a great deal of practice. The latter can be achieved by clinical experience in an emergency department or on an ambulance with a veteran EMT, physician, or nurse observing your technique. It is best to practice under supervision to learn proper techniques and avoid repeating mistakes. You may also team up with a fellow student and take turns "role playing" patients, attempting to extract information from each other, followed by discussion of your effectiveness.

Applying

In the space provided answer your questions.

_____

_____

_____

_____

_____

Evaluating

Were you able to answer all your questions? Yes _____ No _____.
Did the selection give you enough information about the topic? Explain.

_____

_____

_____

_____

_____

Check the accuracy of your answers by finding the specific information in the selection.

STUDENT JOURNAL

List what you have learned about making value judgments.	How would you apply this knowledge to your study or work in the health fields?

Chapter 5

Resolving Conflicts

▼ LEARNING OBJECTIVES

In this chapter you will learn how to

- Analyze conflicts and find appropriate solutions

▼ PREDICTING VOCABULARY

EXERCISE
5-1

Directions: Preview this chapter by finding five words that you recognize but whose precise definition you don't know. Use your background knowledge to write a sentence for each word that predicts the definition of that word.

Word 1: _____

Sentence: _____

_____

Word 2: _____

Sentence: _____

_____

Word 3: _____

Sentence: _____

_____

Word 4: _____

Sentence: _____

_____

Word 5: _____

Sentence: _____

_____

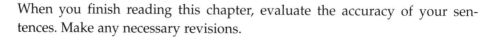

When you finish reading this chapter, evaluate the accuracy of your sentences. Make any necessary revisions.

Revisions

_____

_____

_____

_____

_____

_____

_____

_____

Example 5–1

Read the following about Val's conflict. Her quandary will be referred to throughout this chapter.

Val is a 48-year-old medical assistant working for Dr. Phinius Phlox in his private practice. Dr. Phlox is a busy internist. He sees many adult patients daily and works long hours each day. Even though he is so busy, Dr. Phlox tries to find time to do good works in his community. Val loves most things about her job. While rearing a family, Val went back to school to learn to be a medical assistant. Although it was not easy for her at the time, she is glad she made the sacrifice now that she has found such a fine career. This is Val's second job. When she finished training, she got her first job working in a pediatrician's office. She was unhappy about the distance she had to travel, the weekend hours she had to work, and the noisiness of the babies and children. When she learned of the opening at Dr. Phlox's office, she was thrilled. Not only is she working with adults, but also the office is just minutes from her house and she is not required to work weekends. Dr. Phlox works in a middle-sized medical building. Many types of doctors work in the building. During the 10 years that Dr. Phlox has been located there, he has made many good friends among his professional colleagues. Likewise, Val, in the 6 years she has been working for Dr. Phlox, has made many friends of the nurses and medical assistants who work for the neighboring doctors. Having friends is very important for Val. In addition to being close to Dr. Phlox, she is treated like a member of his family. She has many friends with whom she can take lunch and coffee breaks. Val is appreciative that she has found such stimulating and rewarding work with Dr. Phlox.

Lately, however, dark clouds have been gathering on Val's job horizon. Two months ago, Dr. Peony, a new radiologist from next door, stopped by and asked Val to give Dr. Phlox an envelope when he returned from lunch. After Dr. Peony left, Val could not help noticing that the poorly sealed envelope contained several 20 dollar bills. Although Val was not initially concerned, she began to feel uneasy when this happened every week. She knew that Dr. Phlox liked and respected Dr. Peony and made numerous referrals to her for x-rays and other similar tests. Val began to suspect that the weekly payments of money had some connection to these referrals. She was in a quandary. While Val understood that what the doctors were doing might be illegal, she knew that confronting either of them might put her in jeopardy of losing her job. However, if she ignored the situation, she would feel terrible being part of this potential illegal mess and worried that if the doctors were caught, she would be considered an accomplice since she took the money each time and knowingly handed it to Dr. Phlox. Val felt that she must resolve this terrible conflict immediately.

E X E R C I S E
5–2

Directions: Think about a conflict you may have read about in your health care textbooks or experienced in your personal life or at work. Describe this conflict in the space provided.

_____

_____

_____

_____

_____

_____

_____

_____

_____

_____

▼ UNDERSTANDING CONFLICTS AND SOLUTIONS

Identify conflict → State problem goals → List assumptions → List facts → List limiting factors → Create different solutions

Life being what it is, eventually you may find yourself caught in a dilemma. The dilemma may be as simple as reading contradictory information in your textbooks or may be something more complex that affects your personal life. While avoiding a problem may be out of your control, solving it is not. The first step in resolving any conflict is to understand all the ramifications or details of the problem. Following is a list of the strategies you would use to ensure that you fully grasp the nature of the conflict.

Strategy 1: Identify conflict.

This means that you clearly state the issues that are involved in the conflict. For example, in Val's case, she wrote down the following: "I have a problem. I believe that Dr. Phlox and Dr. Peony are engaging in fee splitting, which is illegal in the medical profession. I have unwittingly become part of the fee splitting by acting as courier of the money."

Strategy 2: State problem goals.

This means that you determine your goal for resolving the conflict. In Val's case, she wanted to stop being part of the apparent fee-splitting scheme and also wanted to get Dr. Phlox to stop engaging in fee splitting.

Strategy 3: List any assumptions, or guesses, you have made about the conflict.

Val realized that she did not have definite proof that fee splitting was going on. Although the money transfer had the appearance of fee splitting, eventually a different explanation might emerge.

Strategy 4: List the actual facts about the conflict.

Val recognized that the two main facts she knew about the situation were that Dr. Phlox was making regular referrals to Dr. Peony and that Dr. Peony was making regular payments to Dr. Phlox.

Strategy 5: List any limiting factors you might experience in the conflict.

This means that you decide what circumstances in the conflict are preventing you from acting. In Val's situation, she was aware that confronting Dr. Phlox with her suspicions would not be easy. She was afraid it would damage their excellent relationship or that she would lose her job.

Strategy 6: Create different solutions.

Val came up with the following ideas for solving her conflict: Talk to Dr. Peony instead of Dr. Phlox. Confront Dr. Phlox and be willing to suffer the consequences. Get professional advice from a lawyer. Do nothing and hope that things would return to normal naturally.

Directions: Refer to Exercise 5–2 in which you wrote about your own conflict. Then fill out the following chart, indicating how you would use the six strategies to understand your conflict better. If you need help, reread how Val used the six strategies for her problem.

EXERCISE 5-3

Strategy 1: Identify conflict.

_____

_____

_____

Strategy 2: State problem goals.

_____

_____

_____

Strategy 3: List assumptions.

_____

_____

_____

Strategy 4: List facts.

_____

_____

_____

Strategy 5: List limiting factors.

_____

_____

_____

Strategy 6: Create different solutions.

_____

_____

_____

▼ INTERPRETING SOLUTIONS

Analyze → Synthesize

Once you have fully understood the various dimensions of your conflict and have thought of some possible solutions, it is time to interpret their feasibility, or the likelihood that they will be effective in solving your dilemma. To do this, you must analyze the different solutions. To analyze the solutions, you must identify the weaknesses and strengths of each of the propositions. Then you must assess how the various solutions will affect you and others involved in the conflict.

Example 5–1

Table 5–1 shows how Val analyzed her solutions according to their strengths, weaknesses, and effects on herself and others.

TABLE 5–1   Val's Analysis of Her Solutions

Solutions	Strengths	Weaknesses	Effects on Me	Effects on Others
Talk to Dr. Peony instead of Dr. Phlox	I may be able to convince Dr. Peony to stop fee splitting without Dr. Phlox knowing about it. This may also stop Dr. Peony from giving me the money so I will no longer be a part of their scheme.	Dr. Peony doesn't know me well and may not feel the need to tell me the truth. She may deny everything and threaten me with a lawsuit. She may tell Dr. Phlox.	It is obviously easier for me to bring this matter up with Dr. Peony than it is with Dr. Phlox. However, I am uncertain how Dr. Peony will react toward my telling her.	Dr. Peony may feel relief that someone else knows about the fee splitting and will see this as an opportunity to stop. Dr. Peony may be livid and threaten to destroy me in order to silence me.
Confront Dr. Phlox and accept consequences	This may encourage Dr. Phlox to stop. Or it may guarantee that I am no longer a part of the fee splitting.	I may lose my valuable friendship with Dr. Phlox. I may lose my job.	I am very anxious because I do not know how Dr. Phlox will react toward me. I dread losing my relationship.	Dr. Phlox may hate me forever and fire me on the spot. He may threaten me with a lawsuit.
Seek professional advice from a lawyer	I will know where I stand legally. I will learn more about fee splitting. I will be taking the first steps in protecting myself legally	I may be told I have insufficient evidence to suspect the doctors of fee splitting.	I will feel relief knowing that someone is helping me with this conflict and giving me the right advice. I am worried about the cost and time this will take.	I may be encouraged to notify the authorities about the fee splitting, which could ruin both doctors. Or if there is not enough evidence, nothing will happen to Drs. Phlox and Peony.
Do nothing	The matter may somehow resolve itself and all can be forgotten.	The conflict will remain unsolved.	I will feel relief if everything blows over without my having to say anything to either doctor. Yet if the fee splitting continues, they may be caught and I would be in trouble also.	The doctors will continue their apparent fee splitting.

Once Val completed her analyses of her different solutions, she saw that none of them was perfect. Yet while she looked over her chart and examined the different components, a new idea occurred to her. Maybe it would be smart if she read up on fee splitting and other legal and ethical matters. She remembered that most of her textbooks began with chapters discussing just these topics. She would begin resolving her conflict by learning more about the issue

What Val did was to analyze her solutions and then synthesize, or recombine, the various ideas to come up with a new solution. In other words, she examined her options and used them as a springboard for creating a new solution. She realized that if she spoke to either doctor, she would have to be very knowledgeable about her accusations. Also, she would have to learn what would count as evidence for fee splitting if she visited a lawyer. And last, she knew she had to do something about the conflict or her anxieties would get the best of her. So by using analysis and synthesis, Val felt that she came up with a reasonable solution to her conflict.

EXERCISE 5-4

Directions: Reread your solutions in Exercise 5–3. Analyze the feasibility of the solutions by filling in each of the components of Table 5–1.

Solution _____

_____

Strengths _____

_____

Weaknesses _____

_____

Effects on Me _____

_____

Effects on Others _____

_____

EXERCISE 5-5

Directions: Reread the chart you filled in for Exercise 5–3. Analyze the feasibility of all your solutions. Use synthesis to come up with a new solution. In the space provided, write down how you now plan to resolve your conflict.

_____

_____

_____

_____

_____

_____

▼ APPLYING THE SOLUTION

Convert solution into action → Implement action

Once you feel you have arrived at a rational solution to your problem, it is time to put your plan to work. If your conflict arose from clashing ideas in your readings, consider writing up your solution as a report. If your conflict arose in your personal or work life, you may want to begin the course of action you decided on. In either instance, applying your solution to your dilemma is what is required at this time.

Since Val had decided to learn more about fee splitting, her course of action led her to the local medical library, where she began to research the topic. One particular passage in a medical assistant's textbook (Kinn, Woods, and Derge, p. 44) caught her attention:

FEE SPLITTING. If a physician accepts payment from another physician solely for the referral of a patient, both are guilty of an unethical practice called **fee splitting.** Fee splitting, whether with another physician, a clinic or laboratory, or a drug company, is unethical.

Val began to realize the seriousness of what she suspected and was now determined to learn more. Continuing her reading in the Kinn et al. text (p. 48), she came upon this passage:

On rare occasions, a medical assistant is faced with a situation in which the physician-employer's conduct appears to violate established ethical standards. Before making any judgments, the medical assistant must be absolutely sure of all the facts and circumstances. If there has in fact been a history of unethical conduct, the medical assistant must then make some decisions. Is it wise to remain under these circumstances or would it be better to seek other employment? This is a difficult decision, particularly if the relationship and employment conditions have been satisfactory and congenial. Will a decision to remain adversely affect future opportunities for employment with another physician?

A medical assistant is not obliged to report questionable actions of the physician or to attempt to change the practice. However, an ethical medical assistant does not wish to participate in the continuance of known substandard practices that may be harmful to patients or that are unlawful.

Val felt tremendous relief when she read this passage. It seemed as though the authors were speaking directly to her situation. One sentence in particular caught her attention: "Before making any judgments, the medical assistant must be absolutely sure of all the facts and circumstances." Val realized that she could never be absolutely sure of all the facts and circumstances. Indeed, there might be some innocent explanation for the cash payments. It became clear that more steps were needed before her conflict would be resolved.

Directions: In the space provided, describe the ways you will apply your solution to resolve your conflict. Indicate if other steps may be necessary.

EXERCISE 5–6

_____

_____

_____

_____

_____

_____

▼ EVALUATING THE SOLUTION

Gather background information → Reason → Choose appropriate alternative

Once you have implemented, or tried out, your solution, you must evaluate or judge the effectiveness of your solution. This evaluation will require that you use two strategies:

• Use background information
• Use reason

Using background knowledge to assist you in evaluating your solution means using all your experience and prior knowledge of the conflict to help you decide if your solution was successful. Using reason to assist you in evaluating your solution means using your intelligence and common sense to help you decide if your solution was successful. This being an imperfect world, you may discover after applying your well-thought-out solution that it was either insufficient for solving your conflict or only partially effective. Then you must choose an appropriate alternative solution to your dilemma.

After Val applied her solution by doing careful research on fee splitting and the medical assistant's obligation for reporting questionable activities, she realized that the answer to her conflict would not be found in a book. Her newly gained knowledge on the topic made her aware of the complexities of the issues and the dangers she might face. She reasoned that the best solution would be to seek the advice of a lawyer, one of the original possibilities she considered when analyzing the dilemma. Using background knowledge and sound reasoning, Val evaluated her current solution and chose an appropriate alternative solution.

Directions: Evaluate the effectiveness of your solution. In the space provided below, fill out the background knowledge and reasoning you used to judge the success of your solution. Indicate if you need to choose an appropriate alternative solution.

Evaluation of Solution

_____

_____

_____

_____

Background Knowledge Used for Evaluation

_____

_____

_____

_____

Reasoning Used for Evaluation

_____

_____

_____

_____

_____

Appropriate Alternative Solution

_____

_____

_____

_____

_____

Conclusion

Val indeed decided to seek the advice of a lawyer and met with Ms. Kessler, a medical attorney. Ms. Kessler told Val that if she suspected professional misconduct and was not acting out of malice, she should make a report to the state health department. This would be the first step in protecting herself. The state health department would then be responsible for investigating the situation and Val could not be sued for making the report. Val would not have to make any reports or be involved with the investigations. The state health department would be in charge.

Val felt she had finally found the right solution to her conflict. It was worth going through the various steps of conflict resolution: understanding conflicts and solutions, interpreting solutions, applying solutions, and evaluating solutions. Val was proud of herself for working through a serious problem and coming up with a satisfying solution.

The state board of health conducted their investigations of Drs. Phlox and Peony without either physician knowing of Val's involvement. The results of their investigations showed that Dr. Peony was giving Dr. Phlox weekly financial contributions for a homeless persons charity that Dr. Phlox headed. They were cleared of any charges of misconduct, and instead both doctors received the keys to the city for their charitable works and contributions. Val recently celebrated her seventh anniversary working with Dr. Phlox.

EXERCISE

5–8

Directions: In the space provided, write the conclusion, or outcome, to your conflict.

_____

_____

_____

_____

_____

CRITICAL READING

Previewing

Preview this selection. Think about what you already know concerning this topic. In the space provided, write what you still need to know.

_____

_____

_____

_____

Questioning

Based on your preview, formulate questions that will help you learn what you still wish to know about the topic. Use the space provided.

_____

_____

_____

_____

Reading

Read the following selection from *The Medical Assistant: Clinical and Administrative* (Kinn et al., 1993).

Council Opinions

The opinions of the Council elaborate and expand the **precepts** in the Principles of Medical Ethics. They are continually updated to encompass developing situations, and they reflect the changing challenges and responsibilities of medicine.

For a fuller appreciation of the ethical issues in medicine, the medical assistant should obtain a copy of the *Current Opinions of the Council* for complete study (Write to: Order Department, OP 122/9, American Medical Association, P.O. Box 10946, Chicago, IL 60610).

Current Opinions, 1989, is presented in nine parts; only a brief summary of these parts appears in the following section.

SUMMARY OF CURRENT OPINIONS OF THE COUNCIL

1.00 Introduction

The introduction explains the terminology used and the relationship between law and ethics. If a physician violates ethical standards involving a breach of *moral* duty or principle, the maximum penalty that the medical society can impose is expulsion. If there is alleged *criminal* conduct relating to the practice of medicine, the medical society is obligated to report it to the appropriate governmental body or state board.

2.00 Social Policy Issues

Abortion. The physician is not prohibited by ethical considerations from performing a lawful abortion in accordance with good medical practice.

Abuse. The discovery that a patient is abusing a child or a parent creates a difficult situation for the doctor's office. The law requires that such abuse be reported. If the physician does not report such abuse in accordance with the law, an added ethical violation is created that may result in continued abuse to the victim.

Allocation of Health Resources. Society must sometimes decide who will receive care when it is not possible to accommodate all who need it. In the case of organ transplantation, for example, there may be several who need the transplant and only one available donor. Who shall be the recipient? Kidney dialysis is another situation where the demand is greater than the supply. This creates a conflict with the physician expected to participate in the decision. The Council opinion is that priority should be given to persons who are most likely to be treated successfully or derive long-term benefit.

Artificial Insemination. **Artificial insemination** requires the informed consent of the woman receiving the artificial insemination and the consent of her husband. In the case of artificial insemination by a donor, the physician is ethically responsible for complete screening of the donor for any defects that may affect the fetus. The identity of the donor is not revealed to the recipient or the resulting child.

Capital Punishment. The physician, being a member of a profession dedicated to preserving life, should not participate in a legally authorized execution, but may certify the death.

Clinical Investigation. Without clinical investigation, there could be no new drugs or procedures. However, all such investigation must follow a competently designed systematic program with due concern for the welfare, safety, and comfort of patients. The physician-patient relationship does exist in clinical investigation, and whenever treatment of the patient is involved, voluntary written consent must be obtained from the patient or the patient's legally authorized representative. Additional restrictions apply when the subject is a minor or a mentally incompetent adult. When participating in the clinical investigation of new drugs and procedures, physicians should show the same concern for the welfare and safety of the person involved as would prevail if the person were a private patient.

Cost. Technologic developments add to the ethical **dilemmas** facing the physician. New expensive treatments are available, and the physician must balance the advantages of these treatments to the patient against their sometimes exorbitant costs.

Genetic Counseling. Genetic counseling and organ transplantation may require personal and ethical decisions concerning the quality of the life that is to be saved.

Organ Donation. The physician should encourage the donation of organs when it is appropriate. However, it is considered unethical to participate in proceedings in which the donor receives payment, except for reimbursement of expenses directly incurred in the removal of the donated organ.

The rights of both the donor and the recipient must be equally protected. In a case involving the transplantation of a vital, single organ, the death of the donor must be determined by a physician other than the recipient's physician.

Quality of Life. Physicians must sometimes decide the fate of a person whose future is dim, such as a deformed newborn or a person of advanced age with many physical problems. The first thought may be the burden to be borne by the family or by society in caring for this person. Ethically, the physician's primary consideration must be what is best for the patient.

Surrogate Mothers. Although **surrogate** motherhood is no longer an isolated entity, many cases are reaching the courts for various reasons. For example, the surrogate may claim bonding to the child and refuse to give it up; the surrogate may decide to have an abortion; or a defective child may be born and neither the surrogate nor the adoptive parents wish to accept custody. The Council does not favor surrogate motherhood as a reproductive alternative for a couple who would otherwise be unable to parent a child because of the many associated concerns.

Withholding or Withdrawing Life-Prolonging Medical Treatment. A physician is committed to *saving life* and *relieving suffering*. Sometimes these two goals are incompatible, and a choice between them must be made. If at all possible, the patient may make this decision. Often, the patient makes his wishes known to a responsible relative or other representative in the event that he or she becomes incapacitated. Patients who live in a state that has "living will" statutes may have some choice if such a will has been established. The living will is a document that states the wishes of that person in the event of a terminal illness. Usually, it is done to prohibit heroic measures being taken in a situation in which the patient would be unable or incompetent to make a decision himself or herself. In the absence of preplanning, the physician must act in the best interest of the patient. If it has been determined beyond a doubt that the patient is permanently unconscious, it is not unethical to cut off life-prolonging treatment.

3.00 Interprofessional Relations

The interprofessional relations of the physician are mostly governed by ethics; however, some legal restrictions do exist. There are state laws that prohibit a physician from aiding and **abetting** an unlicensed person in the practice of medicine or from aiding and abetting a person with a limited license in the provision of services beyond the scope of that license.

The Council addresses the relations of the physician with respect to nurses and specialists, sports medicine and optometry, and involvement with teaching as well as to the referral of patients to other physicians.

If a nurse recognizes or suspects that there is something wrong in a physician's orders, it is the nurse's obligation to report this to the physician. The medical assistant also has this obligation, even if it means risking the displeasure of the physician.

Physicians often refer a patient to another physician for diagnosis or treatment when it is beneficial to the patient. The physician should make these referrals only when he is confident that the patient will receive competent treatment.

In the absence of legal restrictions, a physician is free to choose whom to serve. However, even though the physician may limit his practice, he cannot choose to neglect a patient already in his care.

The sports physician must keep in mind that his professional responsibility at a sporting event is to protect the health and safety of the participants, with his judgment being governed only by medical considerations.

An ophthalmologist may employ an optometrist as ancillary personnel to assist him or her, provided that the optometrist is identified to patients as an optometrist. If the physician does not employ an optometrist, he or she may send a patient to a qualified optometrist for optometric services. Of course, the physician would be ethically remiss if, before doing so, he or she did not ensure that there was an absence of any medical reason for his patient's complaint; the physician would be equally remiss if he or she referred a patient without having made a medical evaluation of the patient's condition.

4.00 Hospital Relations

Most practicing physicians have staff privileges at one or more hospitals. Guidelines for the physician-hospital relationship are developed in this section and include the following:

- It is considered unethical for a physician to charge a separate fee for the routine, nonmedical services performed in admitting a patient to a hospital.
- The physician may ethically bill a patient for services rendered the patient by a **resident** under the physician's personal observation, direction, and supervision, if the physician assumes responsibility for the services.
- The granting of hospital privileges should be based on the training, competence, and experience of the applicant.
- **Compulsory** assessments should not be a condition of granting medical staff membership or privileges.

5.00 Confidentiality, Advertising, and Communications Media Relations

There are no restrictions on advertising by physicians except those that can be specifically justified to protect the public from **deceptive** practices. Standards regarding advertising and publicity have been liberalized over the years, but any advertisement or publicity must be true and not misleading. Testimonials of patients, for instance, should not be used in advertising, as they are difficult, if not impossible, to verify or measure by objective standards. The physician can safely include information of educational background, fees, available credit, and any other nondeceptive information, but statements regarding the quality of medical services are highly subjective and difficult to verify.

HMOs routinely seek members through advertising. Physicians who practice in such prepaid plans must abide by the same principles of ethics as do other physicians. Any deceptive advertising—for example, any that would be misleading to patients or prospective subscribers—is unethical.

Although information regarding some patients, such as celebrities and politicians, may be considered "news," the physician may not discuss a patient's condition with the press without authorization from the patient or the patient's lawful representative. The physician may release only authorized information or that which is public knowledge.

Certain news is a part of the public record. News in this category is known as news in the **public domain** and includes births, deaths, accidents, and police cases.

A statement may be made that the patient was injured by a knife but not that the injury was a result of an assault or accident or that it was self-inflicted. You cannot assert that an action was a suicide or an attempted suicide, nor whether intoxication or drug addiction was involved.

The medical assistant must be aware that only the physician is authorized to release information, and under no circumstances should the medical assistant violate the confidential nature of the physician-patient relationship.

One item of particular interest to the medical assistant is what information may be disclosed by the physician's office to the representatives of insurance companies. It is important to remember at all times that the history, diagnosis, prognosis, and other information acquired during the physician-patient relationship may be disclosed to an insurance company representative *only* if the patient or the patient's lawful representative has consented to the disclosure. You should not even certify that the individual was under the physician's care without the patient's permission. The same restriction applies to discussions with the patient's lawyer.

A physician may testify in court or before a workers' compensation board in any personal injury or related case. In the case of a pre-employment physical examination, although no physician-patient relationship exists, the physician is still bound to the rule of confidentiality; if the physician treats a patient, then the physician-patient relationship is established.

The expanding use of computer technology permits the accumulation and storage of an unlimited amount of medical information. With the use of computers in the physician's office and the employment of computer service organizations, confidentiality becomes more difficult. Detailed guidelines are included in the *Current Opinions*.

6.00 Fees and Charges

It is unethical for a physician to charge or collect an illegal or excessive fee. Illegal charges may occur through ignorance of the law when billing for treatment of Medicaid or Medicare patients. It is a medical assistant's responsibility to keep informed on current regulations and see that they are scrupulously followed.

Fee Splitting. If a physician accepts payment from another physician solely for the referral of a patient, both are guilty of an unethical practice called **fee splitting.** Fee splitting, whether with another physician, a clinic or laboratory, or a drug company, in unethical. The division of practice income among members of a group in joint practice or partnership is determined by the members of the group and is *not* fee splitting.

Lawyers often accept cases on a *contingency* basis, that is, the fee is contingent upon a successful outcome. A physician's fee is always based on the value of the service provided to the patient. Providing care for a fee based upon the success of the outcome would be considered unethical.

Insurance Forms. An attending physician should expect to complete one insurance claim form for the patient without charge. Multiple or complex forms for the same patient may warrant a charge if this is in conformity with local custom.

Interest and Finance Charges. It is entirely appropriate to request that payment be made at the time of treatment, particularly if there has been a past history of late payments. If the patient is notified in advance, it is also proper to add interest or other reasonable charges to delinquent accounts. Advance notice can be accomplished by posting a notice in the reception office or by notations on the billing statements. A more effective approach is the use of a Patient Information Folder that includes billing information; such a folder is provided for every new patient on the initial visit.

7.00 Physician's Records

Notes made by the physician during the course of treating a patient are made for the physician's own use and are considered to be the physician's personal property. They are sometimes used to provide a summary of the patient's treatment to another physician or person at the request of the patient. Original records should never be released except on the physician's retirement or sale of a medical practice.

In some states, a patient is authorized by law to have access to his or her medical records. Health care professionals should familiarize themselves with the laws in their own states. Of primary concern regarding all records is the authorization of the patient before releasing any information, unless the release is required by law.

Records of Physicians on Retirement or Death. There are many reasons that a patient might need access to his health records after a physician retires or dies. The records might be necessary for employment, insurance, litigation, or other reasons. When a physician retires or dies, the patients should be notified and encouraged to find a new physician and to authorize the transfer of their records. Records that are not forwarded to another physician should be retained by a custodian of the records in compliance with any legal requirements.

Sale of a Medical Practice. A physician who retires or the estate of a deceased physician may wish to sell the practice. This sale usually includes the option of taking over the care of the patients who are served by the practice. In such cases, each patient is notified that the practice is being transferred to another physician and that this physician will have custody of the patient's records until such time as the patient may request that the records be sent to another physician.

8.00 Practice Matters

Appointment Charges. May a physician charge for an appointment that is missed or one that was not canceled within a stated time? Yes, but *only* if the patient has been fully advised in advance that such a charge will be made. Discretion should be used, however, in applying such a charge.

Consultation. When a physician refers a patient to a consultant, the referring physician should provide the consultant with the patient's history and any other pertinent information in advance of the consultation. The consultant, in turn, should advise the referring physician of his or her findings and recommendations. On the other hand, if the patient seeks a second opinion from a physician of his own choice, that physician is not obligated to report to the patient's regular physician.

Drugs and Devices: Prescribing. A physician may ethically own or operate a pharmacy or dispense drugs only if such ownership or activity does not result in exploitation of patients. Patients should enjoy the same freedom of choice in deciding who will fill a prescription as they have in choosing a physician. A prescription is an essential part of a patient's medical record, and the patient is entitled to a copy.

Health Facility Ownership by a Physician. A physician may ethically own or have a financial interest in a for-profit hospital or other health care facility such as a freestanding clinic. However, before admitting or referring a patient to that facility, the physician has an ethical obligation to disclose such ownership to the patient. Additionally, the patient's welfare must not be jeopardized by the physician's financial interest; this could happen if the physician unnecessarily hospitalizes or prolongs the patient's stay in the health care facility.

Informed Consent. The patient's right of self-decision can be effectively exercised only if the patient possesses enough information to make an intelligent choice.

Ghost Surgery. The substitution of another surgeon without the patient's consent is called **ghost surgery.** The patient has a right to choose his own physician or surgeon, and to make a substitution without consulting the patient is deceitful and unethical.

Applying

In the space provided, answer your questions.

_____

_____

_____

_____

_____

Evaluating

Were you able to answer all your questions? Yes _____ No _____
Did the selection give you enough information about the topic? Explain.

_____

_____

_____

_____

_____

Check the accuracy of your answers by finding the specific information in the selection.

STUDENT JOURNAL

List what you have learned about resolving conflicts.	How would you apply this knowledge to your study or work in the health fields?

UNIT II

Applying Critical Thinking Skills to Writing

When you are preparing for a career in the allied health fields, you are expected to use writing to complete assignments, learn information, and fulfill job tasks.

You are required to use critical thinking skills in your writing tasks. You may be asked to demonstrate your understanding of course content by writing essays or examination answers. You are expected to use writing to apply the information that you have learned in a course. You might be organizing information on charts or writing letters about new products. You use interpretive thinking skills when you think about the purpose of a writing assignment and how you should organize your information. When you write an evaluation, you are judging or measuring what you have learned and you are thinking about the strengths and weaknesses of the information.

Unit II helps you learn how to apply critical thinking skills to your writing assignments. Chapter 6, Using Patterns of Organization for Clear Writing, helps you learn how to use patterns of organization such as sequence, classification, examples and illustrations, comparison and contrast, cause and effect, and problem solving to collect and outline information. In Chapter 7, Writing Summaries, you will learn the techniques for selecting the most important information in your reading material. Chapter 8, Creating Sound Arguments, shows you how to use deductive and inductive reasoning for logical writing. Chapter 9, Recognizing Fallacies in Writing, explains how to detect and eliminate errors of reasoning in your writing.

Clear writing involves logical thinking. Unit II will give you the critical thinking skills needed to improve your writing tasks in the allied health fields.

Chapter 6

Using Patterns of Organization for Clear Writing

▼ LEARNING OBJECTIVES

In this chapter you learn how to

- Plan your writing
- Gather details
- Use patterns of organization to collect your information
- Use patterns of organization to outline your information

▼ PREDICTING VOCABULARY

Directions: Preview this chapter by finding five words that you recognize but whose precise definition you don't know. Use your background knowledge to write a sentence for each word that predicts the definition of that word.

EXERCISE 6–1

Word 1: _____

Sentence: _____

_____

Word 2: _____

Sentence: _____

_____

Word 3: _____

Sentence: _____

_____

Word 4: _____

Sentence: _____

_____

Word 5: _____

Sentence: _____

_____

When you finish reading this chapter, evaluate the accuracy of your sentences. Make any necessary revisions.

Revisions

_____

_____

_____

_____

_____

_____

_____

▼ UNDERSTANDING USING PATTERNS OF ORGANIZATION FOR CLEAR WRITING

Many students find it difficult to organize information for writing. They can't distinguish between essential information and irrelevant information. These students have to begin with a writing plan, which they can use to organize the topics and details in their writing. A writing plan is made up of the following:

1. **Subject:** *What* is the topic?
2. **Purpose:** *Why* are you writing? Think about your purpose when you plan your organization.
3. **Form:** *How* are you expressing your thoughts? Are you writing a memo, an essay, or a business letter?
4. **Audience:** *Who* are your readers? Are you writing for your teacher, your employer, or yourself?

Use your writing plan to decide how to organize your writing. You have to think about the way to organize your information so that it will best fulfill your purpose. Some common ways to organize your writing are sequence, classification, examples and illustrations, comparison and contrast, cause and effect, and problem solving.

Sequence

The **sequence** pattern helps you write about a process. You should use the sequence pattern when the purpose of your writing is to describe a procedure.

Sequence is a way to describe how something works. Connecting words such as *steps, first, last,* and *later* help your readers follow the steps in your sequence.

Classification

Classification helps you put information into categories. You should use classification when you describe how things are organized and how things are composed. You use the classification pattern when you design charts. Connecting words such as *parts, components, heading,* and *group* help your readers understand the relationship between topics and details in your writing.

Examples and Illustrations

Examples and illustrations are used to back up or support a main idea. When you use examples and illustrations, you carefully select facts and details that are related to your main idea. Signal words such as *for example, explains,* and *kinds of* connect the details you have chosen to explain your main ideas.

Comparison and Contrast

You use **comparison and contrast** to demonstrate how things are alike or different. Connecting words such as *alike, similar, difficult,* and *on the other hand* help your readers remember which details are the same and which are different.

Cause and Effect

You use **cause and effect** to describe reasons and results. You explain why something happens or how something works. Connecting words such as *because, why, result,* and *reasons* help your reader find the cause and result relationships among the details in your writing.

Problem Solving

When you are writing about problem solving, you identify the problem, collect information about the problem, choose the best solution, and prove why your chosen solution was the best. Connecting words such as *wrong, needs, action,* and *plan* help the reader follow the reasoning in your writing.

▼ USING ORGANIZATIONAL PATTERNS TO WRITE AN OUTLINE

Once you have decided how you want to organize your information, you can use your organizational pattern to write an outline. Following is one method of outlining:

Topic Outline

I. Main idea
    A. Important detail
    B. Important detail
       1. Less important detail
       2. Less important detail
    C. Important detail

Another method of outlining is shown in Figure 6–1. Use the method of outlining that best suits your organizational plan.

Example 6–1

Howard was given an assignment to find out why fluoride helps to prevent tooth decay. He used prewriting strategies to create his writing plan. The following is Howard's writing plan and choice of organizational plan:

Subject: Why fluoride helps prevent tooth decay
Purpose: To locate information to answer a question
Form: Report
Audience: Instructor and class

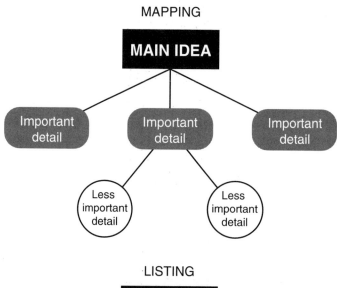

Figure 6–1
One method of outlining

Howard thought about the way to organize his information. The word *why* made him decide to use a cause and effect pattern. He created his outline as a list of causes. The effect, that fluoride helps to prevent tooth decay, was the main idea. He listed several reasons *why* fluoride helps prevent tooth decay. Howard was focused on supporting his main idea, so he chose only details (causes) that backed up the result (effect).

Directions: Read the following assignments. For each assignment, state the pattern of organization that would best fulfill the purpose of the writing plan.

1. Sandy is a receptionist in a doctor's office. She was asked to pull a patient's chart and write a record of the number of visits the patient made to the office for allergy treatments.

   _____

   _____

   _____

2. Maria is studying to be a dental assistant. She was assigned to write about the difference between preparing teeth for bonding and preparing teeth for cleaning.

   _____

   _____

   _____

3. Young-Sun is learning to be a nursing assistant. To prepare for a class on facial fractures, she was asked to list all the facial bones and their exact location.

   _____

   _____

   _____

4. Todd is writing instructions for operating the new computer system. These instructions have to be clear enough for entry-level employees to follow.

   _____

   _____

   _____

5. Felix was asked to write a description of types of chest pain.

   _____

   _____

   _____

6. Heather was assigned to write a research paper on the relationship between smoking and lung cancer.

_____

_____

_____

7. Bryan was typing a paper. When he started to print the paper, half his data was missing. He called the computer company so he could write down their advice on retrieving his data.

_____

_____

_____

8. Kristine was asked to write an evaluation of her chemistry instructor. She liked him personally, but she did not feel that he taught the course well. She is having trouble deciding what to write in the evaluation.

_____

_____

_____

9. James was asked to evaluate two computer systems and to write a memo on the merits and drawbacks of each.

_____

_____

_____

10. George was taking care of a nursing home patient who slipped in the hallway. George's supervisor asked him to write a report explaining why the accident occurred.

_____

_____

_____

▼ INTERPRETING USING PATTERNS OF ORGANIZATION FOR CLEAR WRITING

Once you have created your writing plan and decided on the best way to organize your information to fulfill your purpose, you must decide which facts and details are the right ones to choose for your writing assignment. You have to think about the subject and purpose in your writing plan and select the information that best supports your subject and purpose. Once you've gathered the relevant details and discarded the details that do not support your subject and purpose, you have to decide how to arrange the facts you want to include in your writing.

Example 6-2

Read the following list of factors to consider when deciding what computer system to purchase. An explanation of why certain factors should be discarded follows the list.

Subject: Computer systems
Purpose: Purchasing decisions
Form: Memo
Audience: Employer
Organizational pattern: Comparison and contrast

Details to be compared and contrasted between system A and system B:

1. Cost
2. Size
3. User-friendliness
4. Software package included
5. Age of the sales rep
6. Size of memory
7. Friendliness of sales rep

In the list of details, items 5 and 7 are irrelevant. Neither the age nor the friendliness of the sales rep should be a consideration when making a decision about purchasing a computer system.

Directions: Read the following writing plans, patterns of organization, and lists of details. Decide which details should be discarded based on the writing plans and patterns of organization.

1. **Subject:** Meal planning

   Purpose: To plan a weekly menu for a home health care client

   Form: Chart

   Audience: Home health care workers

   Organizational pattern: Classification

   Details to be selected:

   1. Calories

   2. Proteins

   3. Health requirements of client

   4. Age of dietitian

   5. Balanced diet

2. **Subject:** Cleaning teeth

   Purpose: To describe the procedures for cleaning teeth

Form: Directions

Audience: Dental hygienist

Organizational pattern: Sequence

Details to be selected:

1. Select equipment needed
2. Examination of patient's condition
3. Wear gloves
4. Ask patient about job opportunities
5. Be careful when using sharp instruments

3. **Subject:** Dangers of smoking

   Purpose: To convince smokers to stop

   Form: Lecture

   Audience: Patients with cardiac disease

   Organizational pattern: Cause and effect

   Details to be selected:

   1. Statistics about death rates of smokers
   2. Length of time smoking
   3. Number of cigarettes smoked daily
   4. Coffee consumed daily
   5. Weight of patient

4. **Subject:** Importance of exercise in weight loss

   Purpose: To demonstrate how exercise helps people lose weight

   Form: Report

   Audience: People enrolled in a weight loss program

   Organizational pattern: Comparison and contrast

   Details to be selected:

   1. Compare diets of people in weight loss program.
   2. Compare exercise plans of people in weight loss program.
   3. Compare occupations of people in program.
   4. Compare weight loss by those who have exercised and those who have not.
   5. Compare types of exercises.

5. **Subject:** Household safety

   Purpose: To demonstrate the number of safety hazards in most households

   Form: Pamphlet

   Audience: Mothers of young children

   Organizational pattern: Examples and illustrations

Details to be selected:

1. The number of young children in the neighborhood
2. Wet floors
3. Poisons and household cleaners
4. Sharp-edged tables
5. Medications in unlocked cabinets

▼ APPLYING USING PATTERNS OF ORGANIZATION

Use patterns of organization to create a writing plan.

Directions: Create a writing plan. Choose a pattern of organization. Write an outline based on your writing plan and pattern of organization. Select details that support your subject and purpose.

EXERCISE 6-4

_____

_____

_____

_____

_____

_____

_____

_____

_____

_____

▼ EVALUATING USING PATTERNS OF ORGANIZATION FOR CLEAR WRITING

Use the following checklist to point out strengths and weaknesses of your outline before you proceed to write your first draft.

	Yes	No
1. Did you clearly state your subject?	_____	_____
2. Did you fulfill your purpose?	_____	_____
3. Did you choose a pattern of organization?	_____	_____

4. Did you choose the facts relevant to your subject and purpose?   _____ _____

5. Did you arrange your information so it was easy to follow?   _____ _____

6. Did you use a map, list, or topic outline?   _____ _____

7. Were you objective in choosing your information?   _____ _____

8. Did you recognize the difference between fact and opinion when you gathered your information?   _____ _____

9. Do you feel your outline is clear and accurate?   _____ _____

10. Is your outline organized enough to use in writing your first draft?   _____ _____

EXERCISE 6–5

Directions: Use the preceding checklist to evaluate your writing plan.

_____

_____

_____

_____

_____

_____

_____

_____

_____

_____

_____

_____

CRITICAL READING

Previewing

Preview this selection. Think about what you already know about this topic. In the space provided, write what you still wish to know.

_____

_____

_____

_____

_____

Questioning

Based on your preview, formulate questions that will help you learn what you still wish to know about the topic.

_____

_____

_____

_____

_____

_____

Reading

Read the following selection from *EMT Prehospital Care* (Henry and Stapleton, pp. 680-681).

Introduction

The Emergency Medical Services Act of 1973 outlined seven disease-specific categories around which EMS systems would be designed. Because the government recognized the seriousness of behavioral emergencies, they were included as one of the categories. Caring for patients with behavioral disorders is an area of medicine that is highly subjective, especially for those not specifically trained in psychiatry. Therefore, the standards and guidelines for prehospital care are necessarily general in nature.

There is probably no other area of medicine where the need for careful judgment and experience is more valuable or where there is a greater danger of displaying an inappropriate bias or reacting negatively to patients. This chapter serves as an introduction to one of the most complex areas an EMT will encounter.

Behavioral emergencies can be generally categorized by the type of behavior displayed, such as rage, anxiety, or an attempt at suicide, or by the cause of the behavior, for example, psychosis, hypoglycemia, or head trauma. Behavioral emergencies do not always occur in isolation; many times there will be an emotional component superimposed on an acute organic illness. This chapter covers the magnitude of the problem, types of behavior, their causes, and evaluation and treatment.

The Scope of the Problem

The medical profession often focuses its greatest attention on diseases and conditions that are understandable, measurable, and treatable, such as heart attacks and pneumonia. EMTs also receive most of their training on medical and traumatic conditions. It is easy for EMTs to get the impression that heart attacks are "real" problems and that behavioral problems are not as important. However, this is not true; behavioral emergencies present a great challenge and require a great deal of professionalism and compassion.

Morbidity and mortality statistics suggest that behavioral disorders are of major significance. Depression is said to be present in at least 5% of the population in the United States, with 10 to 20% of adults experiencing at least one episode of clinical depression at some time during their lives. It is estimated that 60% of patients seen by health professionals have underlying emotional disturbances that either cause or contribute to the reason for their visit. Depression is the most common mental disorder in elderly patients. Suicide is the tenth leading cause of death in the United States. About 25,000 people kill themselves each year. The rate of suicide in men over age 65 is at least three times that of the general population; more than 10,000 persons over age 60 kill themselves each year. A young person attempts suicide every 90 seconds in the United States, and another is successful every 90 minutes. From 1950 to 1980, the suicide rate in the adolescent age group tripled. In fact, the death rate for the 15- to 24-year-old age group was the only one in which the overall death rate increased from 1950 to 1980, in large part because of suicide. Significantly, a large percentage of these suicide victims sought medical attention prior to the suicide. In many people, suicidal intentions and depression can be readily treated—if the diagnosis is made.

Medical professionals tend to discount symptoms in people who are difficult, demanding, angry, hysterical, intoxicated, or "crazy." This is an ordinary human reaction, but one that leads to dangerous medical judgment. It is unquestionable that many physical diseases present with behavioral manifestations and that many behavioral problems present with physical complaints. It must remain the goal of all health care personnel to diagnose and treat, and not to judge, discount the potential seriousness of a complaint, or (easier said than done!) become angry with a difficult patient. Remember that it is a natural tendency to discredit the importance of symptoms in people who are emotionally distraught. The interaction between the EMT and the patient often occurs in a highly charged atmosphere, where a person is intensely concerned about his or her well being, anxiety levels are high, and multiple distractions in the environment can interfere with successful care of the patient.

Principles of Communication

General Guidelines

Although individual situations demand different types of interaction, and each EMT has a unique style, there are some general guidelines for communicating with patients and families that are useful.

Focus. Focus your attention directly on the patient, and maintain eye contact. Conversation between EMTs that is directed away from the patient may upset some patients and anger others.

Develop Contact with the Patient. Introduce yourself, informing the patient that you are an EMT and explaining your function.

Tell the Truth. Although you may wish to limit what you say, speak truthfully and do not falsely reassure the patient. If you do not know the answer to a question, admit "I don't know."

Communicate Effectively. Do not use medical terminology the patient may not understand, but on the other hand, do not talk down to the patient.

Use Effective Body Language. The EMT's body posture and gestures should be calm and nonthreatening. An aggressive "body language" can be frightening to the patient.

Speak Clearly. Speak slowly, clearly, and distinctly. With the patient who is hard of hearing, this may require a louder voice; however, avoid shouting, which may frighten the patient.

Explain Treatments. Explain to the patient what you are going to do prior to doing it.

Use the Patient's Name. Use the patient's proper name. Do not refer to a patient as "mom" or "dear." Referring to patients who are your seniors by the first name can be interpreted as being disrespectful. Also, trying to be the patient's "pal" or to "be cool" with the patient is inappropriate and phony. The novice EMT may believe such an approach may be more persuasive with the patient or may make it easier to enlist the patient's cooperation. However, professional demeanor will be much more effective and much less likely to precipitate a scene in which the patient refuses to cooperate.

Allow for Response. The patient should be allowed ample time to respond to questions and not be rushed. This requires expert judgment by the EMT, who must balance the time allowed for the patient to talk against the urgent need to stabilize the patient.

Be Helpful and Considerate. Be aware of the patient's comfort. Is the patient cold? Is he or she in a comfortable position (if it is safe to reposition the patient)? Should a friend or family member accompany the patient?

Look Beneath the Surface. Try to sense the concerns and meanings beneath the patient's words. People call for an ambulance for a reason. A patient who states that he just needs his cardiac medications renewed may have been suffering from chest pain all night but may not tell the EMT this. Patients may deny their symptoms, but be alert when they have a sudden interest in keeping a clinic appointment, refilling medications, or wanting a "checkup."

Be Professional. Maintain a professional and calm demeanor at all times. Do not show anger or personalize a patient's negative remarks. Many people deal with stress and illness by becoming angry, making inappropriate remarks, or hurling insults. This is really just as much a part of the patient's "illness" as is the chest pain or shortness of breath. During times of stress, patients may not have the emotional strength or maturity to show appreciation for the EMT's efforts. Thus, do not be disappointed by the patient who is hostile toward you while you are putting forth your best efforts. The EMT must always be at his or her professional best, even when the job is a "thankless" one.

Anticipate Problems with Communication. Is the patient oriented, angered, hard of hearing, scared? What does the patient expect to happen? If there is resistance to your efforts, why?

Assume Understanding. Always assume that the patient can understand what you are saying, even if it appears that he or she cannot. Avoid inappropriate remarks, and do not talk about the patient as if he or she is not there. It is common, for example, for stroke victims to be unable to speak but to be able to understand everything that is being said.

Applying

In the space provided answer your questions.

_____

_____

_____

_____

_____

Evaluating

Were you able to answer all your questions? Yes _____ No _____. Did the selection give you enough information about the topic? Explain.

_____

_____

_____

_____

_____

Check the accuracy of your answers by finding the specific information in the selection.

STUDENT JOURNAL

List what you have learned about using patterns of organization for clear writing.	How would you apply this knowledge to your study or work in the health fields?

Chapter 7

Writing Summaries

▼ LEARNING OBJECTIVES

In this chapter you will learn how to
- Reduce lengthy articles to their essential ideas by writing summaries

▼ PREDICTING VOCABULARY

Directions: Preview this chapter by finding five words that you recognize but whose precise definition you don't know. Use your background knowledge to write a sentence for each word that predicts the definition of that word.

Word 1: _____

Sentence: _____

_____

Word 2: _____

Sentence: _____

_____

Word 3: _____

Sentence: _____

_____

Word 4: _____

Sentence: _____

_____

Word 5: _____

Sentence: _____

_____

When you finish reading this chapter, evaluate the accuracy of your sentences. Make any necessary revisions.

Revisions

_____

_____

_____

_____

_____

_____

_____

▼ UNDERSTANDING SUMMARY WRITING

A goal for all your writing should be to communicate your ideas clearly to your readers. Regardless of what form your writing takes—research paper, letter, memo, chart, lab report, or patient history—your objective is to convey your thoughts to your audience. When you compose a summary, you are creating a special type of writing that is excellent for all subjects.

Writing a summary not only furthers the goal of clear communication but also helps you learn. To write a summary, you must monitor or be aware of whether you are understanding the article you are to summarize. When you write a summary, you are reducing lengthy articles to important ideas. Summary writing therefore teaches you to focus on important ideas and to write them concisely. When you write a summary, you are rephrasing or substituting your words for the author's words. To rephrase the author's words, you must understand what was written. Summary writing therefore tests whether you comprehend the written material that you are condensing. Learning to write summaries will improve your writing, reading, and critical thinking.

Directions: In the space provided, respond to the following statement: Summary writing is an aid for learning. Explain.

EXERCISE 7–2

_____

_____

_____

_____

There are many ways you can write a summary. The most basic approach is to write in time order. A frame for a time order summary would look like the following.

TIME ORDER SUMMARY FRAME

First this happened in the article. _____

Then this happened in the article. _____

Then this happened in the article. _____

Finally this happened in the article. _____

When you are writing a time order summary, you are using the same format as the article. You are restating the important ideas in the same order that they appeared in the article.

A slightly more complex summary is a visual mapping summary. Figure 7–1 illustrates four ways of drawing a visual mapping summary.

Like the time order summary, the visual mapping summary is concerned only with important ideas. Instead of being in narrative or story form, however, the visual mapping summary is written in diagram form. The visual mapping summary shows how certain important details are related to certain main ideas.

The most abstract type of summary is a chart that shows the more complex relationships among the important ideas in the article. Following are frames of three summary charts.

CAUSE AND EFFECT SUMMARY CHART FRAME

Cause

Important idea 1
Important idea 2

Effect

Important idea 1
Important idea 2

COMPARISON AND CONTRAST SUMMARY CHART FRAME

Comparison

Important idea 1
Important idea 2

Contrast

Important idea 1
Important idea 2

PROBLEM-SOLVING SUMMARY CHART FRAME

Problem

Important idea 1
Important idea 2

Solution

Important idea 1
Important idea 2

The Cause and Effect Summary Chart Frame shows how some important ideas influence other important ideas. The Comparison and Contrast Sum-

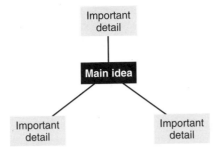

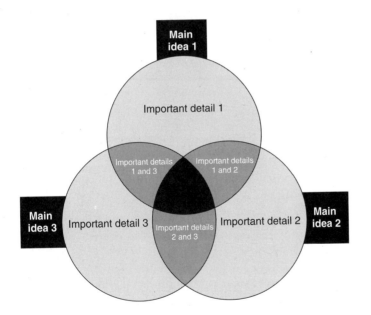

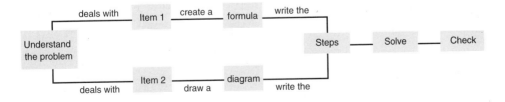

Figure 7–1
Examples of visual mapping summaries.

mary Chart Frame shows the similarities and differences among important ideas. The Problem-Solving Summary Chart Frame shows how some important ideas are the answers to difficult questions. You will use one of these summary chart frames, or comparable ones, depending on how the important ideas are organized in the article you are summarizing.

EXERCISE 7-3

Directions: Answer the following questions in the space provided:

1. What is the purpose of the time order summary?

   _____

   _____

2. What is the purpose of the visual mapping summary?

   _____

   _____

3. What is the purpose of the summary chart?

   _____

   _____

▼ INTERPRETING SUMMARY WRITING

When you write a summary, you have two objectives:

1. Reducing lengthy articles to important ideas
2. Changing the author's words into your own

To accomplish these objectives, learn the following strategies:

- Eliminate less important ideas.
- Eliminate repetitive ideas.
- Combine important ideas into categories, or clusters.
- Create headings for the clusters.
- Write the summary.

Let's take a closer look at each of the preceding strategies for writing summaries.

Eliminate Less Important Ideas

Example 7-1

Read the following passage from *Introduction to Human Anatomy and Physiology* (Solomon, pp. 163-164).

The Conduction System Consists of Specialized Cardiac Muscle

You may have viewed horror films in which a heart beats spookily after being separated from the body of its owner. Some script writers may have rooted their fantasies in a knowledge of cardiac physiology. When removed from the body, the heart can continue to beat for many hours if it is provided with appropriate nutrients and salts. This is possible because the heart has its own specialized conduction system and can beat independently of its nerve supply.

The heart's conduction system is composed of specialized cardiac muscle. This system includes the sinoatrial node, the atrioventricular node, and the atrioventricular bundle (Fig. 7–2). The **sinoatrial (SA) node** is a small mass of specialized muscle in the posterior wall of the right atrium. The SA node is known as the pacemaker of the heart because it automatically excites itself and starts each heartbeat.

The ends of the fibers of the SA node fuse with surrounding ordinary muscle fibers of the atrium so the muscle impulse spreads through the atria, producing atrial contraction. One group of atrial muscle fibers conducts the impulse directly to the **atrioventricular (AV) node,** located in the right atrium along the lower part of the septum. Here, transmission of the impulse is delayed briefly. This delay allows the atria to complete their contraction before the ventricles begin to contract.

From the AV node the muscle impulse spreads into specialized muscle fibers that form the **atrioventricular (AV) bundle** (also called the bundle of His). These large fibers conduct impulses about six times faster than ordinary cardiac muscle fibers. The AV bundle divides into right and left bundles, which extend into the right and left ventricles.

Fibers of the AV bundle end on fibers of ordinary cardiac muscle within the myocardium, so the impulse spreads through the ordinary muscle fibers of the ventricles. Cardiac muscle fibers are joined at their ends by dense bands (intercalated discs). These tight junctions between the muscle cells allow the muscle impulse to pass rapidly from cell to cell. The entire atrium or ventricle contracts as if it were one giant cell.

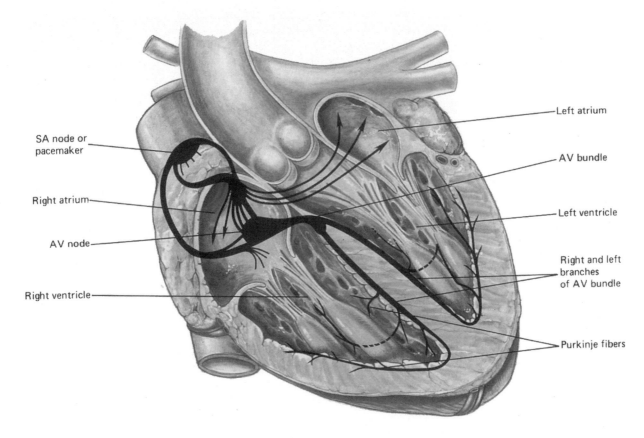

Figure 7–2

The conduction system of the heart. (From Solomon EP: Introduction to human anatomy and physiology. Philadelphia, 1992, WB Saunders, p. 163.)

In summary, the pathway taken by a muscle impulse through the heart is:

SA node → cardiac muscle of atria → AV node → AV bundle → muscle of ventricles

The first step in summary writing is to eliminate less important ideas. To determine what ideas are important and what ideas are not important, look at the heading of the passage. **The Conduction System Consists of Specialized Cardiac Muscle** is the heading for this passage. Turn this heading into a question: **What is the specialized cardiac muscle that makes up the conduction system?** Any fact or idea in the passage that answers this question can be considered an important idea. Any fact or idea that does not directly answer the heading question can be considered unimportant and should be crossed out. If the article you are summarizing does not have headings, create them yourself and make up questions. Figure 7–3 shows the copy one summary writer crossed out because it did not directly answer the heading question.

The Conduction System Consists of Specialized Cardiac Muscle

~~You may have viewed horror films in which a heart beats spookily after being separated from the body of its owner. Some script writers may have rooted their fantasies in a knowledge of cardiac physiology. When removed from the body, the heart can continue to beat for many hours if it is provided with appropriate nutrients and salts. This is possible because~~ the heart has its own specialized conduction system and can beat independently of its nerve supply.

The heart's conduction system is composed of specialized cardiac muscle. This system includes the sinoatrial node, the atrioventricular node, and the atrioventricular bundle (Fig. 7–2). The **sinoatrial (SA) node** is a small mass of specialized muscle in the posterior wall of the right atrium. The SA node is known as the pacemaker of the heart because it automatically excites itself and starts each heartbeat.

Figure 7–3
Annotated section of selection in Example 7–1.

EXERCISE
7–4

Directions: Read the following excerpt from Solomon (p. 179). Turn the heading into a question and write the heading question in the space provided. Then cross out any idea that does not directly answer the heading question.

The Liver Has an Unusual Circulation

As you have seen, blood generally flows from arteries to capillaries and then to veins. The veins conduct the blood back toward the heart. However, the body has a few veins that carry blood to a second set of exchange vessels. Such veins are called **portal veins.** The **hepatic portal vein** delivers blood from the organs of the digestive system to the liver.

Blood is delivered to the intestines by the **mesenteric** (mes"-en-**ter'**-ik) **arteries** and enters capillaries in the intestinal wall. Nutrients are absorbed into these capillaries. Then the blood, rich in nutrients, flows into the **superior mesenteric vein.** This vein empties into the hepatic portal vein, which also receives blood returning from the lower portion of the intestine and from the spleen. The hepatic portal vein conducts blood to the liver, where it gives rise to an extensive network of hepatic sinusoids, exchange vessels somewhat like capillaries.

As blood flows through the sinusoids, liver cells remove nutrients whose concentrations are above homeostatic levels. The hepatic sinusoids deliver blood to the hepatic veins, which leave the liver and empty into the inferior vena cava.

Heading Question _____

_____

Eliminate Repetitive Ideas

Example 7–2

As mentioned earlier, one objective of summary writing is to shorten long articles. A way of achieving this, in addition to eliminating less important ideas, is to eliminate ideas that are mentioned more than once.

Read the following excerpt from *Medical Typing and Transcribing* (Diehl and Fordney, p. 153).

Slang and Vulgar and Inflammatory Remarks

When you are employed in the word processing department of a large clinic or hospital, your supervisor will be able to assist you in the handling of questionable material. Those transcribing for a service whose policy demands verbatim transcription will likewise have a supervisor or director for help. In a private medical office you may, of course, approach the dictator directly. Very few physicians make derogatory or inflammatory remarks, and they may speak in this manner owing to frustrations with their care of the patient. A surgeon may have just lost his or her patient to cancer and tears through the hospital, leaving a path of destruction behind. The "stupid physician" referred to in the dictation he or she leaves behind in your department reflects the frustration in not having a cure. That remark, obviously, is not meant to appear in black and white.

Questionable remarks can reflect on you and your judgment, the physician, the hospital, and the patient. The dictator may refer to patients, patients' families, or other members of the health care team as *stupid, crocks, dumb, lousy surgeons, quacks, "too dumb to know any better,"* and so on. The dictator will usually have forgotten the irritation that precipitated the problem in the first place by the time you transcribe it. Do you transcribe it? Consider these alternatives:

1. Check with your supervisor before transcribing it.
2. Contact the dictator and diplomatically and tactfully ask about it.
3. Make two transcripts, flag the problem, and ask the dictator to make a choice, destroying the original and copies of the rejected transcript (very costly and time-consuming).
4. Leave a blank with a flag that says "I'm sorry but I couldn't quite make out the first three words in paragraph two."

It is better to leave a blank than to type a questionable remark. How you handle the problem will depend on your work situation and your personal contact with the dictator. Consider this example:

"This patient's condition would never have deteriorated to this extent if the nitwit charge nurse on four had brought it to my attention instead of taking it upon herself to practice medicine without a license."

Inflammatory remarks have no place in a medical record and could place innocent people in jeopardy. You were not there when the incident occurred and you have no idea what precipitated this remark, so it would not be your responsibility to edit or delete it. Your responsibility *is* to bring it to the attention of the dictator or supervisor *before* it becomes a permanent part of the patient's medical record.

Your ability to analyze and polish and to proofread effectively and accurately will reflect your professional development. Remember: Follow the protocol available, master the intricacies of English, and become familiar with reference materials and how to use them.

One must remember that medical records are legal documents and while they are vital in the care of patient, they are also vital historically and could be the major protection for the physician in the case of a misunderstanding or a professional liability lawsuit. It is imperative that they be current, accurate, legible, unaltered, and clear.

Figure 7–4 illustrates the same passage, but the summary writer has crossed out ideas that were stated more than once. Be aware that repetitive statements may not appear identical word for word but that they express similar thoughts.

Directions: Read the following excerpt from Diehl and Fordney, p. 273. Then cross out any ideas you believe are repetitive. Remember that the repetitive statements may not be in identical form but will express similar ideas.

PREPARATION OF MISCELLANEOUS MEDICAL REPORTS

A variety of medical reports concerning patients may be transcribed by medical transcriptionists in the Word Processing Department or Medical Records Department of a hospital. On a few occasions, a physician may want his or her private secretary to transcribe some of these reports; and in some medical facilities, the department secretary will do the transcribing. For instance, the Pathology Department may have laboratory reports and autopsy reports transcribed right in the department. Consultation reports may be transcribed in the hospital or physician's office, and medicolegal reports are usually done in the private medical office. Private transcription agencies are prepared to do all kinds of medical typing and transcribing. Since you do not know where you will seek employment, it is necessary for you to be prepared to type these different parts of the medical record.

Reports are sent to consultants who participated in the management of the patient, to insurance companies who wish background information on patients, to third-party carriers to justify bills, to referring physicians, and to the Social Security Administration for assessing a patient for total disability.

Combine Important Ideas into Clusters

Example 7–3

The next step in summary writing requires that you look over the remaining important ideas and cluster, or group together, ideas that relate to one another. The easiest types of relationship to consider for clustering are important ideas that relate to the same general idea. To determine a general idea, review the important ideas you believe to be related and think of a phrase that

Slang and Vulgar and Inflammatory Remarks

When you are employed in the word processing department of a large clinic or hospital, your supervisor will be able to assist you in the handling of questionable material. Those transcribing for a service whose policy demands verbatim transcription will likewise have a supervisor or director for help. In a private medical office you may, of course, approach the dictator directly. Very few physicians make derogatory or inflammatory remarks, and they may speak in this manner owing to frustrations with their care of the patient. ~~A surgeon may have just lost his or her patient to cancer and tears through the hospital, leaving a path of destruction behind. The "stupid physician" referred to in the dictation he or she leaves behind in your department reflects the frustration in not having a cure. That remark, obviously, is not meant to appear in black and white.~~

~~Questionable remarks can reflect on you and your judgment, the physician, the hospital, and the patient. The dictator may refer to patients, patients' families, or other members of the health care team as *stupid, crocks, dumb, lousy surgeons, quacks, "too dumb to know any better,"* and so on. The dictator will usually have forgotten the irritation that precipitated the problem in the first place by the time you transcribe it.~~ Do you transcribe it? Consider these alternatives:

~~1. Check with your supervisor before transcribing it.~~

~~2. Contact the dictator and diplomatically and tactfully ask about it.~~

3. Make two transcripts, flag the problem, and ask the dictator to make a choice, destroying the original and copies of the rejected transcript (very costly and time-consuming).

4. Leave a blank with a flag that says "I'm sorry but I couldn't quite make out the first three words in paragraph two."

~~It is better to leave a blank than to type a questionable remark.~~ How you handle the problem will depend on your work situation and your personal contact with the dictator. Consider this example:

"This patient's condition would never have deteriorated to this extent if the nitwit charge nurse on four had brought it to my attention instead of taking it upon herself to practice medicine without a license."

Inflammatory remarks have no place in a medical record and could place innocent people in jeopardy. You were not there when the incident occurred and you have no idea what precipitated this remark, so it would not be your responsibility to edit or delete it. ~~Your responsibility *is* to bring it to the attention of the dictator or supervisor before it becomes a permanent part of the patient's medical record.~~

Your ability to analyze and polish and to proofread effectively and accurately will reflect your professional development. Remember: Follow the protocol available, master the intricacies of English, and become familiar with reference materials and how to use them.

One must remember that medical records are legal documents and while they are vital historically and could be the major protection for the physician in the case of a misunderstanding or a professional liability lawsuit. It is imperative that they be current, accurate, legible, unaltered, and clear.

Figure 7–4

Annotation of Diehl and Fordney selection in Example 7–4.

would describe all of them. Figure 7–5 illustrates further annotation of the passage from Diehl and Fordney in Example 7–2.

According to the summary writer, the first part of the first paragraph contains important ideas. The points numbered 3 and 4 are also important. Finally, the sentence that starts with "Inflammatory remarks . . ." is considered

---

Slang and Vulgar and Inflammatory Remarks

Important
When you are employed in the word processing department of a large clinic or hospital, your supervisor will be able to assist you in the handling of questionable material. Those transcribing for a service whose policy demands verbatim transcription will likewise have a supervisor or director for help. In a private medical office you may, of course, approach the dictator directly. Very few physicians make derogatory or inflammatory remarks, and they may speak in this manner owing to frustrations with their care of the patient. ~~A surgeon may have just lost his or her patient to cancer and tears through the hospital, leaving a path of destruction behind. The "stupid physician" referred to in the dictation he or she leaves behind in your department reflects the frustration in not having a cure. That remark, obviously, is not meant to appear in black and white.~~

Repetitive
~~Questionable remarks can reflect on you and your judgment, the physician, the hospital, and the patient. The dictator may refer to patients, patients' families, or other members of the health care team as stupid, crocks, dumb, lousy surgeons, quacks, "too dumb to know any better," and so on. The dictator will usually have forgotten the irritation that precipitated the problem in the first place by the time you transcribe it. Do you transcribe it? Consider these alternatives:~~

~~1. Check with your supervisor before transcribing it.~~
~~2. Contact the dictator and diplomatically and tactfully ask about it.~~

Important
3. Make two transcripts, flag the problem, and ask the dictator to make a choice, destroying the original and copies of the rejected transcript (very costly and time-consuming).
4. Leave a blank with a flag that says "I'm sorry but I couldn't quite make out the first three words in paragraph two."

Repetitive
~~It is better to leave a blank than to type a questionable remark.~~ How you handle the problem will depend on your work situation and your personal contact with the dictator. Consider this example:

Not Important
~~"This patient's condition would never have deteriorated to this extent if the nitwit charge nurse on four had brought it to my attention instead of taking it upon herself to practice medicine without a license."~~

Inflammatory remarks have no place in a medical record and could place innocent people in jeopardy. You were not there when the incident occurred and you have no idea what precipitated this remark, so it would not be your responsibility to edit or delete it. ~~Your responsibility is to bring it to the attention of the dictator or supervisor before it becomes a permanent part of the patient's medical record.~~

Not Important
Your ability to analyze and polish and to proofread effectively and accurately will reflect your professional development. Remember: Follow the protocol available, master the intricacies of English, and become familiar with reference materials and how to use them.
One must remember that medical records are legal documents and while they are vital historically and could be the major protection for the physician in the case of a misunderstanding or a professional liability lawsuit. It is imperative that they be current, accurate, legible, unaltered, and clear.

Figure 7–5
Further annotation of Diehl and Fordney selection in Example 7–4.

important. When creating clusters of related ideas, the summary writer thought that part of the first paragraph should be grouped with points 3 and 4. She viewed these important ideas as relating to the general idea of "Alternatives to transcribing questionable materials." So she created the following cluster, putting the important ideas in her own words when applicable. To help the summary writer think of substitute words for the author's, she sometimes had to consult a thesaurus (a dictionary of synonyms). If a word or phrase is a medical or technical term, however, it may be best not to substitute another term for it.

Cluster 1

- Consult with supervisor or director about transcribing questionable material.
- Transcribe two copies, one with the questionable material and one without, and have director decide what copy to use.
- Leave a blank in the transcription where the questionable material is and flag that portion with a note indicating you did not understand the words in the paragraph.

The summary writer then created a second cluster from the important ideas in the paragraph beginning with "Inflammatory remarks. . . ." She thought these important ideas related to the general idea of "Transcriber's responsibility." Note again how she put these important ideas into her own words except when summarizing technical or medical terms.

Cluster 2

- Questionable words do not belong in a medical record.
- However, it is not the responsibility of the transcriber to revise or eliminate the words.

Directions: Read the following selection from Diehl and Fordney, p. 288. Then cross out any unimportant ideas that do not relate to the heading of the passage. Next cross out any repetitive ideas. Finally, in the space provided, group the remaining important ideas into clusters of related ideas.

EXERCISE 7-6

Autopsy Protocols

When a patient dies while in the hospital, permission may be requested from the next of kin to perform an autopsy or postmortem examination of the body to ascertain the exact cause of death. The complete protocol should be made part of the record within 90 days from death. Through autopsies much knowledge has been gained which assists in the diagnosis and treatment of disease. A visual and microscopic examination is done on every organ and related structure. When an organ is removed from a cadaver for purposes of donation, there should be an autopsy report that includes a description of the technique used to remove and prepare or preserve the donated organ. All states have laws that govern autopsies. When someone dies unattended or there is suspicion of a crime (such as violent death, unusual death, self-induced or criminal abortion, homicide, suicide, poisoning, drowning, fire, hanging, stabbing, exposure, starvation, and so forth), an autopsy may be ordered by the court, or it may become the responsibility of the coroner's office to determine the cause of death. The professionals associated with the coroner's office include the following: pathologist, forensic pathologist, forensic dentist, chemist, toxicologist, anesthesiologist, radiologist, odontologist, psychiatrist, and psychologist.

The written record of an autopsy is generally referred to as an autopsy protocol. In pathology, there are five forms: the narrative (in story form), the numerical (by the numbers), pictorial (hand drawings or anatomical forms), protocols based on sentence completion and multiple-choice selection, and problem-oriented protocols (a supplement to the Problem-Oriented Medical Record System).

Frequently a hospital autopsy protocol will contain the clinical history, which is a brief resume of the patient's medical history and course in the hospital prior to demise. It will include the pathological diagnosis made at autopsy, a report of final summary, and the gross anatomy findings (visual examination of the organs of the body before any tissues are removed for preparation and examination). There will also be a microscopic examination (an examination of the particular organs through the microscope). An epicrisis or final pathological diagnosis is given at the end of the protocol. This is a critical analysis (actual finding) or discussion of the cause of disease after its termination.

_____

_____

_____

_____

_____

_____

_____

_____

_____

_____

Create Headings for the Clusters

Example 7–4

As discussed in Example 7–3, to cluster the important ideas that remain after you eliminated the unimportant and repetitive ideas, think of a general idea or phrase to describe each related group of important ideas. Use these general ideas that you formulated as headings for the clusters. The use of headings serves two purposes. First, the headings act as a check to see if you logically grouped the important details in the right clusters. If you are having a hard time thinking of a heading, it may be that your cluster contains unrelated ideas. You may need to create more or different clusters. Second, the headings act as a handle for organizing the ideas when it comes time to write the actual summary. Putting headings on your clusters makes the process of writing summaries more efficient.

Refer to Figure 7–5 and reread the general ideas the summary writer used to create the clusters in that example. She would use those general ideas as headings for the two clusters.

Directions: In the space provided, write the general ideas you made for your clusters. These general ideas will serve as headings for your clusters of important ideas.

EXERCISE
7–7

_____

_____

_____

_____

_____

Write the Summary

Example 7–5

At this point in the summary process you have eliminated unimportant and repetitive ideas, grouped the important ideas around a general idea, and created headings for the clusters. It is now time to write the summary. To write the summary, you will have to order the clusters in a logical pattern. To determine the logical pattern, reread the article and decide on the pattern of organization the author used (see Chapter 6). Let's consider the clusters and headings from Figure 7–5.

Cluster 1. Heading—Alternatives to Transcribing Questionable Materials
- Consult with the supervisor or director about transcribing questionable material.
- Transcribe two copies, one with the questionable material and one without, and have the director decide what copy to use.
- Leave a blank in the transcription where the questionable material is and flag that portion with a note indicating you did not understand the words in the paragraph.

Cluster 2. Heading—Transcriber's Responsibility
- Questionable words do not belong in a medical record.
- However, it is not the responsibility of the transcriber to revise or eliminate the words.

After the summary writer reread the article, she decided that the article described a problem and gave the solution. She therefore felt it would be best to write the summary following the problem-solving pattern of organization. With the problem-solving pattern of organization, she felt that Cluster 2 described the problem and Cluster 1 described the solution. So she rearranged these two clusters. Once the summary writer reordered the clusters, she reviewed the important ideas and rewrote them in the sequence she wanted to use in the summary. The results looked like the following:

Heading—Transcriber's Responsibility
- Questionable words do not belong in a medical record.
- However, it is not the responsibility of the transcriber to revise or eliminate the words.

Heading—Alternatives to Transcribing Questionable Materials
- Consult with the supervisor or director about transcribing questionable material.
- Leave a blank in the transcription where the questionable material is and flag that portion with a note indicating you did not understand the words in the paragraph.
- Transcribe two copies, one with the questionable material and one without, and have the director decide what copy to use.

Note that in the <u>Transcriber's Responsibility</u> cluster, the summary writer kept the same order of important ideas as she had originally. However, in the <u>Alternatives to Transcribing Questionable Materials</u> cluster, she reordered the last two important ideas. Since the summary writer spent time beforehand organizing her ideas and rephrasing the author's words, writing the summary was a simple task. Here is what the finished summary looked like:

> At times, it may be the transcriber's responsibility to decide whether or not to transcribe questionable material. While questionable words do not belong in medical records, it is not the responsibility of the transcriber to revise or eliminate these words.
>
> There are, however, alternatives to transcribing questionable materials. First, the transcriber can consult with the supervisor or director about transcribing questionable material. Second, the transcriber can leave a blank in the transcription where the questionable material is and flag that portion with a note indicating that the words in the paragraph were not understood. Last, the transcriber can make two copies, one with the questionable material and one without, and have the director decide what copy to use.

7–8

Directions: Reread the article in Exercise 7–6. Decide on the pattern of organization. In the space provided, reorder your clusters and the important ideas within each cluster from Exercises 7–6 and 7–7 to reflect the pattern of organization and the sequence you want for the important ideas in the summary. In the following space, write your summary following the plan of the newly rearranged ideas from each cluster.

Reordered Clusters: _____

_____

_____

_____

_____

_____

_____

_____

_____

_____

_____

_____

Summary: _____

_____

_____

_____

_____

_____

_____

_____

_____

_____

_____

_____

▼ APPLYING SUMMARY WRITING

Directions: Following is an article from _Feline Behavior: A Guide for Veterinarians_ (Beaver, pp. 1-4). Read the article and prepare to write a summary by following the strategies below:

- **Eliminate less important ideas.** Read the headings of each section, make heading questions, and cross out any ideas that do not answer these heading questions.
- **Eliminate repetitive ideas.** Remember that repetitive ideas may not be in identical form but will express similar ideas. Cross out the repetitive ideas.

- **Combine important ideas into clusters.** Create each cluster around a general idea. Write your clusters on a separate piece of paper.
- **Create headings for the clusters.** Use your general ideas for your cluster headings. Write the headings next to each cluster.
- **Write the summary.** Reread the article to determine the pattern of organization. Reorder the clusters and important ideas. Rephrase the author's words, using a thesaurus if necessary. Write the summary as a time order summary, visual mapping summary, or summary chart in the space below.

_____

_____

_____

_____

_____

_____

_____

_____

_____

_____

_____

_____

_____

_____

_____

_____

_____

_____

_____

_____

_____

HISTORY OF FELINE DEVELOPMENT

Earliest Origins of the Cat

Down through the ages we have had a curious relationship with the cat. More inconsistent than our relationship with any other domestic animal, it has nurtured the behavior of the modern cat.

The earliest known ancestors of the Felidae date back between 10 million and 45 million years. Carnivores are believed to have shared at that time a common forest-dwelling ancestor: the Miacidae. The cat was derived from a later subdivision, the *Dinictis*. We do not know when the cat was first considered domesticated or which of the wild cats are its ancestors. What is recorded is that by 1600 B.C., cats were domesticated in Egypt. Most authorities agree that the modern cat, *Felis catus*, is derived from *Felis libyca*, the Kaffir cat (also known as the small African bush cat, the African wild cat, or the Caffre cat), which was numerous in Egypt at that time.

The role played by the European wild cat *Felis silvestris* in the development of the modern cat is uncertain. Some contend that *F. silvestris* (formerly called *F. catus*) was crossed with the Egyptian cat to produce the modern *F. catus* (formerly called *F. domestica*), whereas others give behavioral, cultural, and physical reasons to refute this theory. A recent theory is that the two wild types are actually subspecies (*F. silvestris silvestris* and *F. silvestris libyca*), since domestic and wild have identical karyotypes. Molecular studies show a close lineage between the domestic cat and four wild cats, including *F. libyca*.

Spread of the Cat from Ancient Egypt

In ancient Egypt the cat initially was kept to control the rodent population on farms and in granaries. Later the cat also was used to fish and to hunt and retrieve wild birds. As time passed, the cat became associated with religion. Bastet (also called Bast, Bassett), the cat goddess, daughter of the sun god Re, represented the fertility of plants and women as well as good health. As Bastet became the primary goddess, the cat became a prized animal—legally protected; mourned at death by its owner, who showed his grief by shaving off his eyebrows; and mummified for burial in special cemeteries.

The range of the domesticated cat expanded slowly, possibly because of tight export restrictions, which limited emigration to the cat's own ingenuity. Merchants and soldiers eventually introduced *F. catus* to Asia and Europe, so that between A.D. 300 and 500, the cat reached Britain. The correlation between water trade routes and the existence of feline populations shows that water posed no problem to migration; the cats probably traveled by ship, coming and going as they pleased.

Because Muhammad's favorite animal was the cat, it has always enjoyed favor in Islamic countries. Islamic teachings include specific references to punishment for the harsh treatment of cats and other animals. The treatment this animal received from Christians, however, has had a more profound effect on its behavioral development. When introduced into Europe, the cat was believed to have protected the Christ child in the stable from the Devil's mouse. As time passed, the independent nature of the cat and its prominent eyes led to its association with Diana, the moon goddess. Legend has it that she created the cat to mock the sun god Apollo. This association of the cat with the moon led to the connection of the cat with the Devil and witchcraft. During the Middle Ages, not only were vast numbers of cats exterminated, but the same fate was met by people who showed compassion for them. When the European Crusaders returned around A.D. 1600, they brought with them an invasion of the brown rat, the bubonic plague, and a gradual reacceptance of the only effective rat control method—the cat. Introduction into America came in the seventeenth century, probably because the cat served as the principal method of rodent control on British vessels bound for the New World. Along with the cat, however, came the witchcraft cult.

When Pasteur discovered in the 1800s that bacteria spread diseases, people became extremely conscious of cleanliness. By another twist of fate, the cat came to be considered the only clean animal and was allowed in food markets, acquiring a position of favor by merchants.

Domestication of the Cat

Domestication requires several generations of selective breeding to produce physiological, morphological, and behavioral changes. For *F. catus* this process has been unique. Except for the cat, breeding during domestication of most animals had been done by selection of behavioral characteristics, primarily to increase gentleness. The cat, however, was first brought into the home for religious reasons, not utilitarian ones. Because cats followed the urbanization of human populations, mating was a matter of proximity rather than of human selection. Not only was it difficult to control mating in cats, but the religious connotation prohibited selective breeding. The actual date of domestication varies from 100 B.C. to as early as 7000 B.C., and several authorities imply that even now the cat is not fully domesticated because it can revert to total self-sufficiency. The first recorded planned feline breeding did not occur until A.D. 999, at the Japanese Imperial Palace. It soon became fashionable in that country to control cat matings and environments. But mice subsequently devastated the silkworm industry, so that by 1602, Japanese cats were released from these controls.

During the time the cat fell from favor and met with mass extermination in Europe, selective breeding was not practiced. Even with the Crusaders helping the cat return to favor, the prevailing attitude was one of tolerance rather than of full acceptance. Historically, then, it took many years before the cat achieved a position whereby the behavioral characteristics desired in a domesticated animal could be developed by selective breeding.

▼ EVALUATING SUMMARY WRITING

As you have probably figured out by now, summary writing is a complicated process that requires skill. To write good summaries, you must have a great deal of practice. You should not expect to write a perfect summary the first time. It may take many efforts or revisions before you write your best summary. Remember that writing a summary is like any other type of writing: it is a process that requires many attempts before you get it right.

One way to evaluate if you are on target with your summary writing is to fill out a checklist like the one below. If your answers are mostly yes, you know you are writing a good summary. If your answers are mostly no, you may need to redo the areas in which you answered no and revise your summary. Look over your summary from Exercise 7–9 and recall the actual process of writing that summary. Then fill in the checklist in the following exercise.

Did I . . .	Yes	No
read the article well?	_____	_____
eliminate unimportant ideas?	_____	_____
eliminate repetitive ideas?	_____	_____
formulate general ideas that describe all the important ideas?	_____	_____
cluster the important ideas that relate to the same general idea?	_____	_____
create headings for the clusters?	_____	_____
determine the pattern of organization of the article?	_____	_____
reorder the clusters based on the pattern of organization?	_____	_____
sequence the important ideas in each cluster by the way I want to write them in the summary?	_____	_____
follow this new reordered plan of important ideas when I wrote the summary?	_____	_____
rephrase the author's words into my own, except for medical or technical terms?	_____	_____
use a thesaurus for help in rephrasing the author's words?	_____	_____
write a summary that is considerably briefer than the article?	_____	_____

CRITICAL READING

Previewing

Preview this selection. Think about what you already know about this topic. In the space provided, write what you still wish to know.

_____

_____

_____

_____

_____

_____

_____

_____

Questioning

Based on your preview, formulate questions that will help you learn what you still wish to know about the topic. Use the space provided.

_____

_____

_____

_____

_____

_____

_____

_____

Reading

Read the following selection.

Manuscript Preparation

In most cases, the medical assistant's tasks in connection with the preparation of a talk or a **manuscript** for publication are mainly mechanical; the doctor is responsible for the actual writing. However, since many physicians ask their medical assistants to serve in the capacity of editorial assistants and to smooth out and actually edit their copy before submitting it for publication, a basic understanding of the style, format, and characteristics of medical papers is helpful.

Writing Style. Each medical journal has its own style for publishing papers. The individual hoping to publish in a specific journal should request a copy of the journal's guidelines for manuscripts in advance and then prepare the manuscript accordingly in order to minimize editorial changes. However, there are certain fairly uniform procedures to be followed in the preparation of a manuscript to be submitted for publication.

A good medical paper must present established new facts, modes, or practices; principles of value; results of suitable original research; or a review of facts on a subject from which the reader can draw a legitimate conclusion. The subject should be limited to a definite area or problem before writing is begun, and the purpose should be determined in advance.

The typical medical article begins with an introductory section outlining the nature of the material or problem to be covered, follows with actual discussion of the subject, and concludes with a summary in which conclusions are usually noted in numeric form. The format for case reports is somewhat similar. Case reports based on clinical information should be written clearly in smooth narrative style and should not read like a collection of telegraphic notes. There should be a clear presentation of the sequence of events. A brief abstract may appear at the beginning or end of any article. This summary should be rigidly condensed and should contain the deductions as well as clearly reflect the author's viewpoint. Only the actual conclusions reached should be numbered.

The writing in a scientific paper should be simple and straightforward. Excess words should be ruthlessly pared from the article. Grammatical construction must facilitate direct, clear expression. The paper should be well organized and proceed smoothly from beginning to end in a direct fashion. Slang, **colloquialisms,** personal allusions, and reminiscences should generally be avoided in papers for publication, although they are often acceptable and add a friendly tone to a paper to be delivered in person before a medical meeting.

Typing the Manuscript. Many **drafts** of a paper may be made before the final copy. Using an electronic word processor or computer can greatly reduce the laborious retyping of manuscripts, but the author may still want a printout of each revision. Sometimes different colors of paper are used to distinguish between each draft. Double- or triple-space drafts to allow plenty of room for revisions by the author.

Revising the Manuscript. An important step in the preparation of any manuscript is a careful revision of copy. This is a duty sometimes delegated to the secretary or medical assistant. Revisions should be made with these specific objectives in mind:

- Organization
- Accuracy
- Content
- Conciseness
- Correct sentence and grammatic construction
- Clarity and smoothness

Check for correct spelling, using a medical dictionary as well as a standard dictionary.

Preparing Final Copy. Use good-quality 8½"× 11" white paper. Type on one side of the paper only. Double-space the copy, allowing a margin of at least 1 inch at each side and at the bottom. Double-spacing provides space for the editor who receives the manuscript to make corrections or insert instructions for the printer. Unless otherwise instructed, number each page in the upper right-hand corner.

The original manuscript is submitted to the publisher, and the author should retain one or more copies. If the manuscript is on disk or tape, one printout is sufficient to retain in the file.

Footnotes. When a paper is based on a study of the writing of others, it is necessary to acknowledge the sources used. In medical and scientific papers, **footnotes** usually provide exact references to sources of material. Forms of footnotes differ slightly, depending on the style of the particular periodical, but in general a footnote contains the following:

- Author's name
- Title of the work cited
- Facts of publication
- Exact page from which the citation was taken

The first time a book or article is mentioned in a footnote, all the information about publication should appear in the footnote; after that, references to the same source can be shortened to the author's last name and the page number cited. When a periodical is concerned, a later reference need contain only the author's name, the journal name, and the page number.

Detailed information about footnote preparation can be obtained from *The Chicago Manual of Style* or one of several published reference manuals for office workers.

Final Bibliography. All scientific papers should carry a complete bibliography of source materials. List only those sources that directly pertain to the paper and that were used in its preparation. The form of bibliographies is fairly uniform.

A periodical listing includes:

- Author's name and initials
- Title of the article
- Name of the periodical
- Volume number
- Pages cited
- Date of publication

A book reference includes:

- Author's name and initials
- Title of the book
- Edition (only after the first edition)
- Place of publication
- Name of the publisher
- Year of publication

Bibliographies may be arranged alphabetically according to authors' names or numerically as the references appear in the text. Whatever form and punctuation are used should be consistent throughout the entire listing (Table 7–1).

Illustrations. All drawings, photographs, and other illustrative material submitted with a manuscript should be placed on separate sheets and keyed to the manuscript. In other words, illustrations should be numbered, and indications should be noted in the manuscript as to where each illustration should be place. Do not include such materials in the body of the manuscript. The explanation of the drawing or illustration should appear in a caption, or **legend.**

Glossy black and white photographs reproduce best. Captions for photos should be typed on separated sheets or may be attached with rubber cement below the photo. On the back of the photograph, the author's name and the number of the illustration should be penciled lightly. Do not use paper clips on photos. Credit lines should be given for copyrighted or commercial photos or illustrations. If x-ray films are submitted, make sure the prints are shiny; indicate on the back where they may be cropped, but leave localizing landmarks.

Charts and line drawings must be carefully prepared in order to achieve good reproduction. Such drawings preferably should be done with India or black ink on heavy white bond paper. Charts should be condensed and simplified as much as possible. Letters and identifying numerals can be placed on the face of the chart with the explanation in the legend below.

Tables should be typewritten on separate sheets in a uniform style; each table should be numbered consecutively and have a descriptive heading.

Mailing the Manuscript. Generally, manuscripts should not be folded but should be mailed flat in a large envelope. Sometimes a paper of fewer than four pages can be folded twice and mailed in a regular business envelope, or a manuscript of four to eight

TABLE 7–1 Abbreviations Used in Manuscript Preparation

Abbreviation	Meaning
cf.	compare
e.g.	for example
et al.	and other people
ibid.	in the same place
i.e.	that is
loc. cit.	in the place cited
op. cit.	in the work cited
sic	intentionally so written
q.v.	which see

pages can be folded once and mailed in a 6 × 9 inch envelope. A letter stating that the manuscript is being submitted for publication should be included. Photos and illustrations should be mailed flat, between sheets of protective cardboard.

Proofreading. A paper accepted for publication will be set in type, and proofs of the article will usually be returned by the editor to the author for checking. Since changes in a manuscript once it is set in type are costly, revisions should be limited to correction of errors and minor changes.

If possible, work as a team when checking **galley proofs,** with one person holding the proofs and the other person reading from the original copy. Check for typographic errors, omitted lines and words, and so forth. When correcting proofs, use a different-colored pencil from the one used by the proofreader on the publication. Corrections should be entered in the margins of the proof, next to the line with the error to be corrected. A knowledge of proofreader's marks is helpful (Fig. 7–6).

One corrected set of galley proofs should be returned to the editor, and one set of proofs should be retained by the author. If a second set of proofs is sent later, check the first corrected set against the second set to make sure all corrections have been made.

Indexing. Often it is necessary to provide an index for a long paper or a book. An author and subject index can be made from page proofs. One system for indexing is to use slips of paper or 3 × 5 inch cards. Each index entry is listed on a separate card, or slip; this sim-

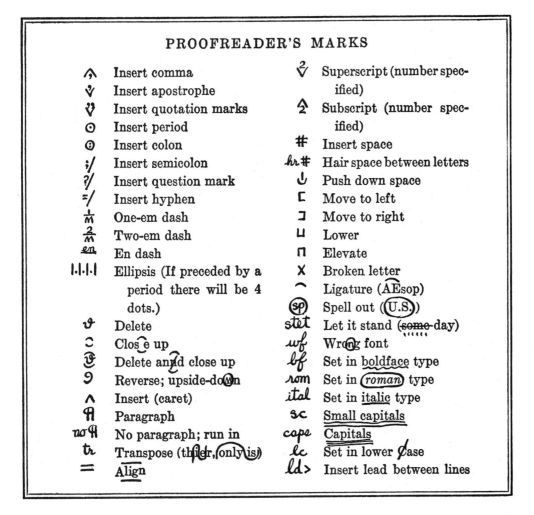

Figure 7-6
Proofreader's marks.

plifies alphabetizing under major headings later. The whole index can then be typed from the alphabetized cards. Manuscripts prepared by computer can be indexed quickly and accurately with the necessary software.

Reprints. At the time an article is set in type, the physician should order all reprints needed, since type is often destroyed after the original press run. Most doctors send copies of their articles to colleagues, to physicians who have evidenced an interest in their work, and to hospitals and teaching institutions with which they have had contact. They probably maintain a card file of names and addresses of those to whom they want to send reprints.

The medical assistant generally handles the ordering of the reprints, which may be as many as 500 copies or more. The order should be adequate to cover any future needs. Addresses in the card file should be checked from time to time in the *American Medical Directory* or by scanning membership and request lists. Some record of reprint mailing should be kept, and acknowledgments should be checked. A person who does not acknowledge two or three reprints should be taken off the mailing list.

An enclosure care, printed in advance, is sent by some authors with a copy of the reprint. Others prefer to enclose a short letter stating that the reprint is a complimentary copy.

Speeches. Not all papers are intended for publication. Some are prepared for presentation before medical and scientific meetings. Speeches should be typed and double-spaced; in some offices, a jumbo or magnatype machine is used so that the speech is easy to read. Special large-type elements, such as the IBM Orator, are available for single-element or daisy wheel typewriters.

At the bottom of each page, in the lower righthand corner, type the first two or three words that appear at the beginning of the next page. The final draft of the paper should be carefully checked for typographic errors.

At large meetings, a speaker is usually allotted from 10 to 20 minutes to present a paper; at county society and small meetings, the speaker may have from 30 minutes to an hour for the presentation. Check in advance to find out exactly how much time will be allowed. The doctor or the medical assistant should time the speech. On the average, it takes about 2 minutes to read a page of copy on which there are about 200 to 250 words. If slides or other illustrations are planned, arrangements for showing this material must be made in advance and the necessary time allowed.

Applying

In the space provided, answer your questions.

_____

_____

_____

_____

_____

_____

Evaluating

Were you able to answer all your questions? Yes _____ No _____
Check the accuracy of your answers by locating the specific information in the selection.

Did the selection give you enough information about the topic? Explain.

_____

_____

_____

_____

_____

_____

_____

_____

STUDENT JOURNAL

List what you have learned about writing summaries.	How would you apply this knowledge to your study or work in the health fields?

<h1>Chapter 8</h1>

<h1>Creating Sound Arguments</h1>

▼ LEARNING OBJECTIVES

In this chapter you will learn how to
- Use inductive and deductive reasoning to organize facts for logical writing

▼ PREDICTING VOCABULARY

Directions: Preview this chapter by finding five words that you recognize but whose precise definition you don't know. Use your background knowledge to write a sentence for each word that predicts the definition of that word.

Word 1: _____

Sentence: _____

_____

Word 2: _____

Sentence: _____

_____

Word 3: _____

Sentence: _____

_____

Word 4: _____

Sentence: _____

_____

Word 5: _____

Sentence: _____

_____

When you finish reading this chapter, evaluate the accuracy of your sentences. Make any necessary revisions.

Revisions

_____

_____

_____

_____

_____

_____

_____

_____

_____

▼ UNDERSTANDING SOUND ARGUMENTS

When Prospero, a first-year student studying veterinary technology, had to write his first paper, he was stymied. Although he had chosen an interesting topic, "The Grief Process in Pet Loss," and had written many facts down on note cards, he had no clue how to organize his ideas into a logically written paper. Prospero spent a great deal of valuable time staring at his note cards, wishing he knew how to arrange the facts in a sound, coherent manner. If Prospero had known about **inductive and deductive reasoning,** the task of writing his first paper for his veterinary technician program would have been much simpler.

Inductive Reasoning

Inductive reasoning is the process of investigation and discovery. Consider, for example, the job of a criminal detective. It is her responsibility to solve the mystery of the crime by drawing a conclusion from the clues. These clues, the wrench in the billiard room or the bloody footprints on the carpet, are pieces of the puzzle the detective must put together to form a complete picture of the criminal act. The detective uses inductive reasoning, looking at specific pieces of evidence to come to a general understanding of who committed the crime. Consequently, inductive reasoning can be described as going from the specific to the general.

Similarly a physician uses inductive reasoning when diagnosing a patient's illness. When consulting with the doctor, the patient describes the specific symptoms. After considering these symptoms, the physician is able to figure out the nature of the patient's illness and provide her with a diagnosis. Like the detective, the doctor is putting together pieces of the puzzle to create the whole picture. The physician is using inductive reasoning.

Inductive reasoning therefore is a process of investigation or discovery in which you use specific clues, symptoms, or ideas to form a solution, diagnosis, or conclusion. You are using particular details to help you develop a main idea.

Directions: In the space provided, draw a simple diagram describing inductive reasoning.

Deductive Reasoning

Deductive reasoning is the process of relating general principles or abstract ideas to specific examples or cases. Health care professionals use deductive reasoning to test hypotheses, apply the steps of a procedure, or determine the relationship of cause and effect. To determine the course of treatment for a patient after a diagnosis, the doctor uses deductive reasoning. For example, the doctor judges that her patient is suffering from a bad cold. She must choose the correct treatment: chicken soup, fruit juices, antibiotics, aspirin, over-the-counter cold preparations, or nothing. The doctor uses deductive reasoning to go from her understanding of the general principles of the cold to her specific recommendation for treatment.

Similarly, deductive reasoning is used at the crime scene. The coroner, or person responsible for determining time of death in a murder, uses deductive reasoning. The coroner uses specific principles to establish the time the person was murdered. The coroner knows the rate at which a body loses a specific amount of heat. Once the temperature of the body is taken, the coroner can deduce how long the person has been dead.

Deductive reasoning can be considered the opposite process to inductive reasoning because you reason from the specific to the general. You are using a general principle or abstract idea to help you find specific examples. You are moving from the main idea to particular details that relate to the main idea.

Directions: In the space provided, put in your own words the process of deductive reasoning.

▼ INTERPRETING SOUND ARGUMENTS

Whether you use inductive reasoning or deductive reasoning as a basis for organizing the ideas in your paper, you are using sound logic to present your facts. When you use inductive reasoning as a means of organizing your ideas, you are organizing the facts so you will be able to conclude the paper with a general interpretation of these facts. When you use deductive reasoning as a means of organizing your ideas, you are organizing the facts so that you will be able to use the facts to solve a problem, to demonstrate the application of a principle, or to test an hypothesis introduced at the beginning of the paper. In both instances, you are ordering the ideas in your paper logically.

After learning about inductive and deductive reasoning, Prospero was beginning to get a handle on how to order the ideas for his paper on the grief process in pet loss. However, he had to decide which of these two processes would be more suitable for his ideas. Prospero felt that creating visual mappings of his ideas in an inductive and deductive manner would be helpful. He could then use the mapping as an outline for his paper. He knew that if he decided to use inductive reasoning for his paper, the facts would have to be mapped in a way that would allow him eventually to draw a conclusion or interpret them. Prospero tried the styles of visual mapping for inductive reasoning illustrated in Figure 8–1.

Prospero knew that if he decided to arrange his ideas deductively, the facts would have to be mapped in a way that would allow him to present the principles, problems, or theories first and then link them to specific cases and examples. Prospero tried the visual mapping in Figure 8–2 as a means of organizing his ideas deductively:

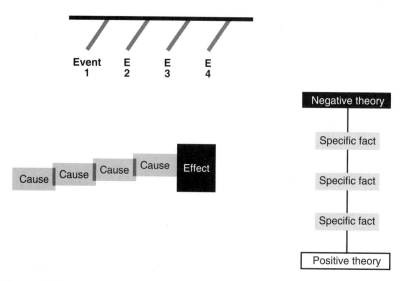

Figure 8–1

Examples of inductive visual mappings.

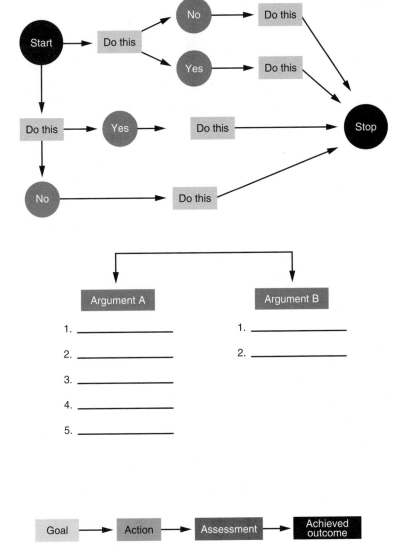

Figure 8–2
Examples of deductive visual mappings.

Example 8–1

Here are some of the ideas Prospero has for his paper on the grief process in pet loss* and examples of an inductive visual mapping and deductive visual mapping he made using these ideas (Figure 8–3).

Stage 1: Denial; Goal—to accept the reality of the loss
Stage 2: Bargaining; Goal—to experience the pain of grief
Stage 3: Anger; Goal—to adjust to an environment in which the deceased is missing
Stage 4: Depression; Goal—to withdraw emotional energy and reinvest it in another relationship
Stage 5: Acceptance

*Data from McCurnin D M: Clinical textbook for veterinary technicians, ed. 3, Philadelphia, WB Saunders, p. 524.

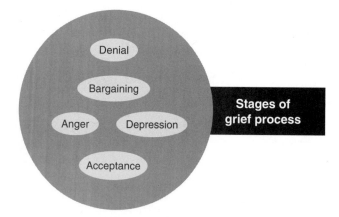

Inductive mapping of grief process

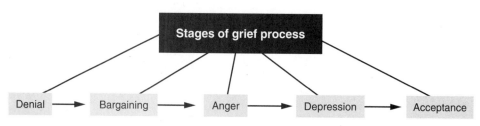

Deductive mapping of grief process

Figure 8–3
Examples of visual mappings Prospero made for his paper.

EXERCISE
8–4

Directions:

Step 1. In the space provided, write down a title for a topic with which you are familiar.

_____

_____

_____

_____

Step 2. On the following lines, write down five facts about this topic.

1._____

2._____

3._____

4._____

5._____

Step 3. Draw one example of an inductive visual mapping of your ideas from step 2. Remember that you are reasoning from the specific to the general. Refer to Figure 8–1 if necessary.

Step 4. Draw one example of a deductive visual mapping of your ideas from step 2. Remember that you are reasoning from the general to the specific. Refer to Figure 8–2 if necessary.

▼ APPLYING SOUND ARGUMENTS

Prospero was now getting ready to write his paper. Since he had ample time, he decided to write two short rough drafts, one organized for the inductive process and one organized for the deductive process. Let's take a closer look at how he wrote each of the drafts.

Example 8–3

Prospero had learned that inductive reasoning begins with the specific and proceeds to the general. To apply this notion to his paper topic "The Grief Process in Pet Loss," Prospero realized he had to begin his paragraph with behavior and symptoms of grief over pet loss. Then he had to specify the principles of the corresponding stages in the grief process. Using his inductive visual mapping as an outline, he wrote the following paragraph.

Two months ago, Judy's twenty-year-old cat, Daisy, died of kidney failure. At the grocery store, she found herself still buying cat food. She constantly prayed for a miracle that would restore her cat to her. She called up her veterinarian twice to blame him for neglect and inappropriate treatment. Her sleeping and eating patterns were disrupted. However, after consulting with the veterinary technician and her family doctor, Judy began to feel normal again. She learned that she was experiencing the normal stages of grief: denial, bargaining, anger, depression, and, finally, acceptance.

EXERCISE 8-5

Directions: Refer to your inductive visual mapping from Exercise 8–4, step 3. Use these ideas to write a paragraph using inductive reasoning as a means of organizing the facts. Remember to go from the specific to the general.

_____

_____

_____

_____

_____

_____

_____

_____

_____

_____

Example 8–4

Prospero also learned that he could organize the facts in his paper deductively. This means that the paragraphs begin with a general idea and proceed to specific examples. When he wrote his paragraph, Prospero had to begin with a statement of the stages of grief and then specify the application of the various stages. Here is how Prospero wrote his paragraph using his deductive visual mapping as an outline.

Through research, we have come to understand the process of bereavement and to recognize each of the five successive stages: denial, bargaining, anger, depression, and, finally, acceptance. This knowledge has allowed Judy to recover from her pet loss. When Daisy, Judy's twenty-year-old cat, died of kidney failure, Judy could not recognize her own behavior. At the grocery store, she found herself still buying cat food. She was constantly praying for a miracle that would restore her cat to her. She called up her veterinarian twice to blame him for neglect and inappropriate treatment. Her eating and sleeping patterns were disrupted. However, as time went by and Judy consulted with the veterinary technician and her family doctor, she began to feel better and accept the loss of her cat.

Directions: Refer to your deductive visual mapping from Exercise 8–4, step 4. Write a paragraph using deductive reasoning as a means of organizing the facts. Remember to go from the general principle to specific examples.

EXERCISE **8–6**

_____

_____

_____

_____

_____

_____

_____

_____

▼ EVALUATING SOUND ARGUMENTS

Now that Prospero has two models for his paper, his final step is to evaluate whether inductive or deductive reasoning will suit his organizational purposes better. He remembers that you use inductive reasoning when you want to draw a conclusion. He has also learned that you use deductive reasoning to understand cause and effect, test a hypothesis, or solve a problem. Prospero's purpose for writing this paper is to understand what happens in the grief process for a person who has experienced the loss of a pet. He sees this as a cause and effect problem, so he has decided to use deductive reasoning.

To evaluate whether to use inductive or deductive reasoning, you must determine your purpose for writing a paper. Once you are aware of your purpose for writing, you will be able to evaluate easily whether induction or deduction is appropriate for your writing needs.

Directions: Following is a list of reasons for writing a paper. Evaluate whether inductive or deductive reasoning would be most suitable for each reason. Write "I" for inductive or "D" for deductive in the blank line next to each item.

EXERCISE **8–7**

1. Organizing ideas chronologically to understand a trend in history _____

2. Categorizing the traits of different mammals under headings _____

3. Testing the validity of a psychological theory _____

4. Understanding the correct procedures for lifting a patient _____

5. Grouping facts to make a discovery ____

6. Drawing inferences from a pie chart ____

7. Weighing the evidence in a criminal trial ____

8. Recognizing changes in the plot of a novel ____

9. Finding examples to support a theory ____

10. Creating a theory to fit the facts ____

CRITICAL READING

Previewing

Preview this selection. Think about what you already know about this topic. In the space provided, write what you still wish to know.

_____

_____

_____

_____

_____

_____

_____

Questioning

Based on your preview, formulate questions that will help you learn what you still wish to know about the topic. Use the space provided.

_____

_____

_____

_____

_____

_____

Reading

Read the selection.

Pet Loss and the Grief Process

The death of a pet is all too often regarded as a trivial loss by society, perhaps owing in part to the mistaken belief that pets can be easily replaced. There are no socially sanctioned rituals like funerals or memorial services to help grieving pet owners gain support once the bonds between them and their companion animals have been broken. Furthermore, people are rarely granted time off from their jobs in order to care for sick animals or to make arrangements for them after their deaths. Society also does not allow adequate time for mourning the death of a pet. Most people feel pressured to be "back to normal" within a few days of their pet's death in order to avoid being labeled as neurotic, hysterical or overly attached. However, crying, taking time away from work, and wanting to memorialize a pet are healthy responses to the death of a pet. They should not be discouraged, nor should they be judged.

One of the most effective ways for veterinary professionals to assist grieving clients is to educate and reassure them that their feelings and behaviors are normal parts of the grief process.

The Normal Grief Process

As stated earlier, the word process implies movement toward some end or result. In regard to grief, this movement is accomplished by passing through what have been termed stages, phases or tasks. The basic emotional process in pet loss is the same as in human loss. However, veterinary professionals who assist clients are aware of some differences and particulars.

Several models of the grief process can be modified to describe the emotional process that occurs during pet loss. Some important ones are exemplified in Table 8-1. For our purposes, we will use the classic model supplied by Elisabeth Kübler-Ross (1969) and extrapolate for the situations peculiar to pet loss.

Dr. Kübler-Ross was one of the first to work extensively with the dying and their families during the late 1960s. She described the grief process as consisting of five "stages": denial, bargaining, anger, depression, and resolution. She used the stages to describe the passage through grief, but it is helpful to remember that these stages are not a linear odyssey. Although people may travel through the grief process in a straight line, they more often fluctuate between stages, bounce back and forth, and feel the entire gamut of grief within minutes, within days or within months.

TABLE 8–1   Popular Models of the Grief Process

Kübler-Ross	Worden	Rosenberg	Dersheimer
Stages	Tasks	Stages	Phases
Denial	I. To accept the reality of the loss	Denial	Shock
Bargaining	II. To experience the pain of grief	Anger/guilt	Acute grief
Anger	III. To adjust to an environment in which the deceased is missing	Grief	Straightening up the mess
Depression	IV. To withdraw emotional energy and reinvest it in another relationship	Acceptance	Reinvesting and re-engaging in life
Acceptance			

Stage 1: Denial

Denial is a normal defense mechanism that buffers a human being from some unbearable news or reality. It is important to recognize the word "normal" here, as many individuals experiencing denial at the time a poor prognosis is given or during bereavement will seem to all observers to be out of touch with reality. The veterinary staff may wonder whether the client has even heard the veterinarian stating the seriousness of an animal's illness. A client in denial may listen attentively to a diagnosis of cancer with a poor prognosis, but ask only if the toenails can be clipped or if their current flea shampoo is correct. A client informed of the death of their pet while it was hospitalized may chatter on about activities for the weekend. A simple form of denial is exemplified by the client who states repeatedly, "It can't be. I don't believe it."

It is tempting when presented with a client experiencing denial to insist that they recognize the seriousness of the situation. Many veterinarians and veterinary technicians worry that the client does not comprehend or has not heard correctly. There is no harm in repeating oneself to a client in denial. In fact, restating diagnoses, prognoses, treatment plans and particulars is advisable. However, clients in denial will only accept the unbearable reality of the situation when they are ready internally; attempts to push them may backfire, resulting in frustration. Usually, a client will begin to ask appropriate questions about the time they arrive home and may phone the veterinary office. Some may even seem to return to reality before your eyes while those toenails are being attended to. The veterinary professional must feel assured that the client has been told the basic information that needs to be given. Remember, however, that it may not have been fully understood; therefore, always leave the door open for further communication.

Although denial reappears later during the grief process, at that time it is usually of little significance to the veterinary staff. Later-stage denial may be manifested as clients reporting during a phone call or visit that they were sure they had seen their pet that morning, or they had absent-mindedly purchased pet food several weeks or months after their pet's death. Denial is reflected by the client's eyes and demeanor, and by incongruous questions. The veterinary staff should not feel responsibility to "break through" a client's denial. The client will move out of denial, accepting the reality of the situation, when he is ready. The veterinary staff's recognition of the client's denial can prevent impatience and frustration during the veterinary contact.

Soft Paw, a 15-year-old female domestic shorthair cat, is brought into the clinic for vomiting and anorexia that the owner thinks is due to the ingestion of chicken bones. Physical examination reveals Soft Paw to be thin and pale. Further evaluation reveals that Soft Paw is severely anemic due to renal failure. The prognosis is poor.

Soft Paw is owned by a 20-year-old college student named Ashley who found the cat as a kitten. Ashley has owned Soft Paw since she was 5 years old. When told that Soft Paw's problems were not caused by chicken bones but were due to end-stage renal failure Ashley at first did not seem to hear what the doctor had said. A blank stare washed over her face, and for a moment she appeared to be daydreaming. The doctor continued by explaining that there were some treatments that may prolong Soft Paw's life, but they should be considered palliative and not potentially curative. After hearing the doctor's assessment Ashley smiled, picked up her cat and turned to leave. "Thank you for your time today," she said as she turned to leave. "I'll try not to let her get into the chicken bones in the future. Oh, by the way, can you trim Soft Paw's front claws? They are getting kind of long."

Ashley came to the veterinarian's office for what she perceived to be a problem brought on by Soft Paw's dietary indiscretion. Ashley had probably not seen her cat eat chicken bones but was grasping for an explanation for why Soft Paw was vomiting, losing weight and acting lethargic. In all probability, Ashley had been denying that Soft Paw was sick for some time even before making the appointment with the doctor. When the doctor told Ashley the diagnosis her initial reaction appeared to be that of shock. Ashley's shock, seeming not to hear the results of the evaluation, and asking the doctor to perform something seemingly inappropriate like a nail trim is part of denial, the first stage of grief.

When a client like the one presented above is encountered, the veterinary professional must realize that the response is a normal part of the grief process. The conversation up to that point may or may not have been heard, but it certainly has not yet been clearly comprehended. The client will be able to acknowledge the seriousness of the situation only when he or she is ready internally. The veterinary professional should repeat things and not become frustrated or impatient. Clip the nails and call the client at home later for further discussions. At that time the client may be ready to acknowledge the reality of the bad disease, and meaningful discussions concerning treatment options can then occur.

Stage 2: Bargaining

Once the reality of death or impending death is realized, the client may show various impotent attempts to control or to reverse the reality. The client is grappling with the stage of the grief process that Dr. Kübler-Ross called bargaining. During this stage, the client maneuvers personally and privately, possibly praying and negotiating with God for miracles. They might add various herbs and old family remedies to food. Children behave like little angels, hoping to be rewarded with a reversal of bad news. The veterinary staff may be subject to various inquiries by the client at this stage, such as, "Have you ever heard of avocado in the food? I read that it may reverse cancer." It is while bargaining that a pet owner may also request permission to obtain a second (and sometimes third, fourth or fifth) opinion. Bargaining during terminal illness rarely results in harm to the patient, and veterinary staff should reassure themselves of their clients' normality. Be compassionate and when possible answer their questions. Help clients to understand that this stage of grief is normal.

Bargaining after death has occurred may go on without the knowledge of the veterinary professionals involved. Seeking to "replace" the lost animal without grieving at all is a form of bargaining. Many pet owners seek a new pet too soon, and they purchase the same species, the same color, and name them the same or a similar name. Leaving dishes or the dead pet's belongings down for an obviously unusual length of time is another subtle form of bargaining. Through bargaining the client is unconsciously attempting to control or subvert the grief process.

It is important to recognize bargaining as part of the normal grief process. The veterinary professionals who understand the stages of bargaining and denial will avoid frustration in their attempts to provide quality patient care and client service.

> **Three days after the euthanasia of his Doberman "Saber," Ron came into the clinic to pay his bill. After reviewing the bill, he asked to speak to the veterinarian who was busy at the time. Maggie, the technician, led Ron to an examination room and then inquired as to how he had been doing. Ron told her that he had not been sleeping well because of dreams of Saber. He stated that the dreams were pleasant, but he would awaken hoping that Saber's death had been a nightmare. He said, "Sometimes I'll keep my eyes closed for an extra ten seconds and pray that she's come back, somehow, healthy and happy. But of course, it never works." In addition, he said, "I want to see Dr. Roberts today because I can't stop thinking about Saber's treatment. I know Dr. Roberts is the best vet around, and I'm grateful to him for being so kind to me and Saber. But I feel like maybe something more could have been done."**
>
> **Ron met with Dr. Roberts for only a few minutes. During this time Maggie was asked to bring tissues to the room. As Maggie handed him a tissue, Ron said tearfully, "I looked at the whole record. Even while I was doing it, I realized that no information could bring Saber back to life. For some reason, I had to look anyway. Now, maybe, I can let her go."**
>
> Although Ron understands that Saber died, he feels compelled to try controlling the situation. Childlike and irrational behaviors such as his closing his eyes and wishing or praying that Saber was alive are manifestations of the bargaining stage of grief. Ron's request to view the record might have been viewed by the veterinarian and the technician as challenging or accusatory. Yet Ron was not looking for information which could be damaging, he was hoping again to somehow reverse the illness and death of Saber. Bargaining can be frustrating for veterinary professionals unless they understand and assist the client in working through these irrational attempts to "bring their beloved pet back."

Stage 3: Anger

During the grief process, clients may move in and out of the stage called anger. Clients coping with this stage may exhibit anger in a wide variety of direct or indirect manners.

The anger may be specific or nonspecific in the way that it is directed. Anger may also be exhibited in the form of guilt, which can be defined as anger turned inward.

Anger is a particularly difficult emotion to deal with when a client directs it toward the veterinary professional. Whether or not the client is justified in his stated cause for anger, staff members must use tolerance and patience to avoid responding defensively. Bereaved clients may complain that the illness which resulted in death should have been discovered sooner, should have been treated differently or should not have been allowed to happen. They may complain that their pet died while hospitalized owing to neglect or inappropriate treatment rather than to the tumor revealed by necropsy.

Anger may be apparent in the form of guilt. Clients feeling guilt use language with an abundance of "I should've" statements. They often seek the listening ear of the veterinary professional to ask questions pertinent to absolution from guilt. They may ask whether or not the food they fed their pet could have contributed to the illness or death. They often ask whether or not it was the pesticide in their home or in the shampoo that caused a tumor or cardiac arrest. Clients may believe they allowed their pet to be too active or too fat; others may believe they caused the kidney failure in their cat by feeding insufficient diet. These clients can direct anger at themselves, but frequently they cannot find a specific crime that they committed. When possible, the veterinary professional can assist the client by assuaging their guilt. Reassuring the client that, in your opinion, they did everything possible for their pet, that they did only what they thought would benefit their pet and that they made the right decisions for their pet will relieve much of the client's guilt or anger and assist him in moving through the grief process.

The client showing indirect and nonspecific anger is not as threatening to the veterinary professional as those who direct their anger specifically toward the veterinarian or veterinary technician. The client who is feeling this type of anger may be gruff or rude and generally hard to get along with. Stating that he is angry, he may be at a loss to express with whom or what he is angry. This type of anger is common in American society. These clients yell at the cashiers, waitresses and telephone operators; and they drive their cars with aggressiveness and anger. Giving the angry client an opportunity to express his feelings (ventilation) is an effective way for the veterinary professional to help. At times, all that is needed is for the sensitive veterinary professional to explain that, considering the client's loss, anger is a normal feeling. This explanation gives the client permission to grieve effectively.

Indirect and specific anger in a client is most often exhibited by reluctance to pay the bill. Upon receiving an inquiry by telephone, the client implies that nonpayment is due to anger at treatment by the veterinarian or by the technician, the pet was neglected, that the illness was mistreated or that he (the client) was treated insensitively. Bereavement support can alleviate this client's anger. Listen attentively, state your apologies, if any, and follow up with this client. No admission of mistakes need be made, but the client needs to feel significant and understood.

Although all of the types of anger may be exhibited by one client, it is guilt that may be hardest for the client to relinquish. Yet, direct and specific anger, when justified (or perceived to be justified), is difficult to work through, as well. In continuing to feel guilt and anger, the client avoids letting go of the beloved pet, and the grief process is stymied. Once the client is able to relinquish the guilt or anger, the grief process can continue.

The veterinary professional can assist the client with all types of exhibited anger by taking a mental step back and a deep breath, committing to a nondefensive attitude and simply listening. Take notes if possible and reassure the client of follow up if his anger is directed at veterinary staff. Assuage any guilt if the opportunity arises, and allow the client to ventilate. A few minutes on the phone or in person may salvage a client relationship and go a long way in assisting the client through the grief process.

Honey, a 12-year-old male Poodle, is presented for a second opinion. He has been having seizures for almost a year. They have been occurring more frequently and have been increasing in severity over the past few months. Another veterinarian has told the owner that the diagnosis is epilepsy and that there is nothing further that can be done.

Not wanting to accept that "Honey's" seizures cannot be controlled, Charles, a 40-year-old businessman, takes Honey to another veterinarian for a second opinion. The second veteri-

narian diagnoses the problem as a brain tumor and offers referral to a veterinary school for surgery. While Charles is considering his options, Honey has a severe seizure and dies. Charles calls the second veterinarian to let him know of Honey's death. He refuses to wait for the veterinarian to come to the phone, is rude to the receptionist and hangs up abruptly. Two days later he calls to apologize and expresses feelings of guilt for not bringing Honey to the second veterinarian sooner. He also informs the second veterinarian that he has stopped payment on his check to the first veterinarian. A week later the second veterinarian is contacted by Charles' lawyer inquiring as to his willingness to testify should Charles elect litigation against the first veterinarian for malpractice.

Charles is showing signs of anger. Anger should be recognized as a stage of grief. It can be directed in many ways. In this case Charles' initial anger is nonspecific and indirect, being manifested as rude behavior on the phone. The person taking the phone call and absorbing the brunt of this initial anger should realize that the anger is not personal and is not necessarily directed at him. He should not react defensively but should listen politely and let the client know that he empathizes and understands. Charles later calls to apologize for his behavior and at that time reveals his feelings of guilt at not making up his mind concerning referral sooner and for continuing to take Honey to the first veterinarian for almost a year. Assuring Charles that the short time over which he was thinking over his options had not made a difference may help relieve some of the guilt. Also assuring Charles that the first veterinarian could not have known of the tumor based on the initial signs and that the same course of events was likely even if he had sought a second opinion sooner may also alleviate guilt and prevent further questioning of the initial veterinarian's diagnosis. By stopping payment to the first veterinarian Charles is showing indirect and specific anger. Later the anger is directed specifically at the first veterinarian when Charles seeks the advice of a lawyer concerning the professional conduct of the first veterinarian. Communication between the first veterinarian, the second veterinarian and Charles will probably be necessary for Charles to work through the anger stage of grief.

Stage 4: Depression

The stage of the grief process that is termed depression has also been called "grief." Clients experiencing depression describe their mood as complete, overwhelming sadness, a feeling of "lead in their boots" accompanied by bouts of uncontrollable crying. Intense grief can result in depression, which prohibits a client from functioning normally. Appetite is changed, energy level is lowered, the client withdraws from others and sometimes is unable to go to work. More subtle symptoms of depression include irritability, sleep irregularity, restlessness and inability to concentrate.

The veterinary professional has occasion to recognize depression due to pet loss when follow-up contacts are made with the client. Depression, when severe, usually sets in some time after the loss. Clients with poor social support systems, elderly clients and clients with intense and/or symbolic attachment to the pet may experience worrisome depression. When contacts are made several days or weeks after bereavement, and it is suspected that a client is depressed, referral can be made to a counselor or hotline specializing in pet loss. Although referral sometimes feels awkward, it might be gently phrased as, "I know a person experienced in counseling people who have lost their pets." Again, reassurance that grief is normal is of benefit.

Most clients experience the feeling of being overwhelmed by their emotions because of grief. They state the feeling of being out of control in their emotions. They may also state surprise and worry that they are reacting with such intensity to the death of an animal. They may be embarrassed. It comforts clients when veterinary professionals confide that most pet owners feel and act similarly upon the loss of the pet. Assuring them of your knowledge of their pet's importance as well as your respect for their grief is valuable to them.

Grief must be worked through, not bottled up; thus, it is a process requiring some emotional catharsis. Many clients cry, and some are uninhibited about expressing anger and sadness. They may loudly complain, and they may sob unabashedly. Becoming comfortable with one's own emotions facilitates comfort with others' emotions. It is human and necessary to feel empathy for grieving clients, but it can also be uncomfortable and painful. Separating your own feelings from theirs will allow you to transform empathy into sympathetic gestures that help the client.

Mary Jo, a 64-year-old widow, brings her 3-year-old dog for examination. She states that the young dog, a mixed breed named Boo, is lethargic and just does not seem to be "getting over" the death of her Golden Retriever, Lucky. As she talks with the technician, she states that even though Lucky died a month ago, Boo is depressed all the time. The veterinarian examines Boo, and determines that the dog is in perfect health. Also, Boo wags his tail, strains at the leash, licks the veterinarian and the technician, and appears happy and energetic.

The technician, left alone with Mary Jo for a few minutes, inquires as to how she is feeling in regard to the death of Lucky. Mary Jo begins to cry softly and says, "I just can't stop crying. I miss him so much. I've lost ten pounds, and I just don't feel like doing anything. Sometimes I stay in bed most of the day. I know my friends and my children think I should be over it, and I don't talk with them about it anymore. I feel silly to be still grieving over an animal. I think I dealt with my husband's death better than this."

The technician lets Mary Jo talk about Lucky for many more minutes. Some of the time Mary Jo cries, but much of the time she tells amusing stories and both individuals laugh. Finally, when Mary Jo breaks down into tears again, the technician puts her hand on Mary Jo's shoulder and says, "I understand now why you're still grieving. Lucky was so special to you, and it might take you awhile to grieve. Support and someone to talk to can help. May I provide you with a telephone number of an understanding counselor?"

Three weeks had passed when Mary Jo telephoned the technician. With a new lift in her voice she reported that both she and Boo were doing much better. After talking with a counselor, she found a way to memorialize Lucky, and she cries less each week. "I called because I'm ready to look for a playmate for Boo, and of course, a new friend for me. Do you know of anyone with puppies?'

Without the contact due to Mary Jo's other pet Boo, her depression may have gone unnoticed by the veterinary professionals. Many times clients suffer through the stage of depression feeling very much alone and as if they have nowhere to turn for help. Depression may occur on and off during the entire grief process (as in the client who sobs uncontrollably just after a pet has died) or depression may become more serious later on in the grief process. At that time, support for the bereaved may no longer be available within their circle of friends and family. It is important to follow up on clients who have poor support systems or who are unusually attached to their animals. Referral to professionals can be of great assistance in helping these clients resolve the grief process.

Stage 5: Resolution or Acceptance

The stage of resolution and acceptance is the feeling that everything is okay, normal functioning is restored and emotional energy is reinvested. The dead pet has been "let go of" emotionally. This does not mean that the pet is forgotten but that it has been assigned to a special place in the bereaved individual's heart. New attachments can be made without regret and hesitation. Resolution may come easily for some and may be difficult for others. In general, children reach the stage of acceptance and resolution more quickly and more easily than do adults. As stated previously, the grief process is not linear, and bits of this stage occur with more and more frequency and with longer durations throughout the grief process. Eventually, the client who successfully resolves the grief process feels little, if any, of the first four stages.

The question is often raised whether clients should "replace" an animal before they reach resolution of the grief process. The process itself is highly variable in length. It can be as short as a few weeks to as long as many years. Most pet owners are able to reinvest and reattach to a new pet at any time, but only after they become aware that replacement of their unique loved one is impossible. If companionship, tactile closeness and friendship are desired while grieving, it can be obtained through a new pet. Cautioning and encouraging clients to choose animals somewhat dissimilar to their dead pet can be helpful. Having a new pet forced on the grieving individual who is not ready to reinvest in a new relationship will only end up furthering heartache in both the bereaved and the new pet.

Applying

In the space provided, answer your questions.

_____

_____

_____

_____

_____

_____

_____

Evaluation

Were you able to answer all your questions? Yes _____ No _____
Check the accuracy of your answers by locating the specific information in the
selection.
Did the selection give you enough information about the topic? Explain.

_____

_____

_____

_____

_____

_____

_____

_____

_____

STUDENT JOURNAL

List what you have learned about inductive and deductive reasoning.	How would you apply this knowledge to your study or work in the health fields?

Chapter 9

Recognizing Fallacies in Writing

▼ LEARNING OBJECTIVES

In this chapter you will learn how to

- Recognize three types of fallacies
- Make logical corrections for the fallacies

▼ PREDICTING VOCABULARY

Directions: Preview this chapter by finding five words that you recognize but whose precise definition you don't know. Use your background knowledge to write a sentence for each word that predicts the definition of that word.

EXERCISE 9–1

Word 1: _____

Sentence: _____

_____

Word 2: _____

Sentence: _____

_____

Word 3: _____

Sentence: _____

_____

Word 4: _____

Sentence: _____

_____

Word 5: _____

Sentence: _____

_____

When you finish reading this chapter, evaluate the accuracy of your sentences. Make any necessary revisions.

Revisions

_____

_____

_____

_____

_____

_____

_____

_____

▼ UNDERSTANDING FALLACIES

Carmen was exceedingly disappointed. For one of her classes she had been asked to write a "point of view" paper. Carmen had chosen to write about home health care. In her paper she had taken the position that it is beneficial for society to have the government financially support home health care programs because that service is cheaper than hospitalizing or institutionalizing patients. Carmen worked hard on her paper and felt confident that she had done a good job. However, when she got her paper back, Dr. Jiminez had written on the top sheet that her paper was filled with fallacies. Carmen had no idea what fallacies were. So during her next study session, Carmen went to the school library to do some research.

A fallacy is a mistake in reasoning. Such a mistake usually occurs when the student draws the wrong conclusion about the premise, or evidence, in the argument. As a result, the premise does not support the conclusion and a fallacy occurs. While there are many types of fallacies, some of the more common types follow:

- Begging the question, or circular reasoning
- Cause and effect errors
- Jumping to conclusions

Let's take a closer look at each of these examples of fallacious logic or fallacies.

▼ BEGGING THE QUESTION, OR CIRCULAR REASONING

Begging the question, or circular reasoning, occurs when you come to a conclusion that is logically the same as the evidence or premise of your argument. In other words, you are trying to prove something is true by assuming ahead of time that it is true. For example, consider the following dialogue:

Trixie: Health care students live in the city.
Lester: How do you know that?
Trixie: Because they live in the city.

Trixie is begging the question, or using circular reasoning, because she is proving her point by making the same point.

Now consider this discussion:

Trixie: Health care students live in the city.
Lester: How do you know that?
Trixie: Because they live in New York, Chicago, and Boston.

In this instance, even though Trixie's argument may not be right, she is not begging the question or using circular reasoning.

Not all examples of begging the question or using circular reasoning are as obvious as the preceding one. Read this more complicated example of begging the question or circular reasoning:

Good grades require that you spend 3 hours studying per day, attend all classes, and finish homework assignments on time. Therefore, to be a good student you must spend one eighth of your day studying, be at all your lectures, and hand in all assignments in a timely and regular manner.

Even though these two sentences are not identical, they both state the same ideas. This is another example of begging the question or circular reasoning.

Directions: Below are 10 statements. Cross out any of the statements that are examples of begging the question or circular reasoning.

EXERCISE **9-2**

1. Willie believes that all babies are stupid because babies do not know much.
2. Willie believes that all babies are stupid because they cannot talk or read.
3. Getting too much homework is not helpful to new students because getting too much homework is useless to new students.
4. Getting too much homework is not helpful to new students because getting too much homework does not allow the new student to adjust to a new program.
5. I could not care less if you agreed with me because it does not matter if you agree with me or not.
6. To be a good reader, you must know how to decode new words. Therefore to be an excellent reader you must know now to figure out new words.
7. To be a good reader, you must know how to figure out new words. Therefore, to read well you must know the sounds of vowels and how to break new words into syllables.
8. Education does not end the day you graduate because you keep on learning the rest of your life.
9. Being polite to others is critical because it is important to show good manners to other people.
10. Being polite to others is necessary because it makes people feel positive about you.

▼ CAUSE AND EFFECT ERRORS

A cause is the reason something happens. An effect is the result. Therefore the cause must happen first and then the result follows. This is illustrated by the following sentence:

When the baby cried, the father picked her up.

In this instance, "when the baby cried" is the cause or reason something happened. "(T)he father picked her up" is the effect or happened as a result of the cause. The baby's crying occurred first, and the father's picking her up happened afterward. This is a true and logical cause and effect statement.

Errors with cause and effect statements occur when the statement is inverted or reversed. Consider this example:

The father picked up the baby when she cried.

In this sentence, even though "the father picked up the baby" is written first, it is still the effect or result of the cause, "when she cried." Even though the effect is mentioned first in the sentence, it is still the effect and not the cause. Therefore, to avoid making cause and effect errors, you must do two things:

1. Read or write all cause and effect statements carefully and thoughtfully.
2. Do not assume that the cause will always be in the first part of the statement. Even though logically and in reality the cause happens before the effect, when you write you can switch the order for diversity in sentence structure.

Directions; Below are 10 cause and effect statements. Mark "C" over the part of the statement that is the cause and "E" over the part of the statement that is the effect. Be alert to cause and effect sentences that are inverted or reversed.

1. When the sun came up, the rooster crowed.

2. He failed the exam when he lost his notes.

3. Despite the doctor's good care, the patient died.

4. She made numerous typing errors after drinking a beer at lunch.

5. When the cat lost her favorite toy, she grew restless and anxious.

6. She became head of the unit when her boss retired.

7. He had to retake the patient's blood after he accidentally dropped the tube.

8. If there is sufficient light, the eye sees.

9. The woman's bones will remain strong with the proper intake of calcium.

10. The more calories you ingest, the greater your weight will be.

▼ JUMPING TO CONCLUSION FALLACY

A jumping to conclusion fallacy occurs when you reach a conclusion about **all** members of a category when you have only observed a few examples from that category. A good example of jumping to conclusion fallacy can be found in the following dialogue.

Daughter: Mom, can I have my ears pierced?
Mom: No.
Daughter: But Marianne and Amanda have their ears pierced. Everyone has her ears pierced but me.

In this instance, the daughter is jumping to conclusions when she assumes everyone has her ears pierced when she knows this about only two girls, Marianne and Amanda. To avoid this fallacy, the daughter should have argued that her two best friends have pierced ears. This argument would probably hold more weight with Mom than "everyone is doing it."

Consider this second example:

Two patients who smoke have a hard time getting to their therapist's office on time. The medical receptionist now thinks that all patients who smoke will turn up late for their appointment.

Again, this is a good example of the medical receptionist jumping to conclusions. Instead of thinking that all patients who smoke come late, she should realize that it is only these two patients and not all smokers who are not prompt.

Directions: Below are five jumping to conclusion statements. In the space provided, rewrite the statement so it is no longer a fallacy of jumping to conclusions.

EXERCISE 9-4

1. I did well in high school math. College math will be too easy for me.

_____

_____

2. She is good at training all animals. Since she was 6, she has had two well-trained cats.

_____

_____

3. Since there are no homeless people in my town, there must be no homeless people in my entire state.

_____

_____

4. The 10-year-old dental patient has never had a cavity His teeth are well cared for so he will never have any.

_____

_____

5. For the last two visits, I had to wait over an hour for my appointment. This time I will arrive at the doctor's an hour later than my scheduled appointment.

_____

_____

▼ INTERPRETING FALLACIES

After Carmen did her research and learned more about fallacies, she was ready to go back and look for the fallacies in her paper. Here is a portion of the paper Carmen wrote about home health care workers.

It is beneficial for the federal and state governments to financially support home health care workers because it is advantageous for the governments to do so. Many millions of dollars will be saved if the elderly and chronically ill can be kept out of hospitals and nursing homes. At present, it costs $180,000 annually to maintain an elderly person in a nursing home. This same patient can be cared for at home with a daily full-time home health care worker for $30,000. Thus, if all elderly patients everywhere could be kept at home, much money would be saved.

It is a wise idea to support the home health care project any way we can because it is smart to do so. Patients gain by home health care. Because of home health care, the patients can persevere in much of their regular daily routine. They are more comfortable physically when they remain in familiar surroundings. Patients are more content emotionally because they are not isolated from family and friends. Home health care is helpful for patients because it helps people in many ways.

One example of good home health care concerned 80-year-old Maimie. She was diagnosed as suffering from chronic bronchitis and asthma. It was becoming increasingly more difficult for Maimie to live independently. Her family considered either a nursing home or home health care for her. After considering both the costs and Maimie's emotional well-being, the family chose home health care. A worker now visits her four days a week and helps with bathing, shopping, housekeeping, and minor medical procedures. Maimie is still able to visit with her friends and family and on good days go out to restaurants, movies, and card games. Consequently, patients with pulmonary problems would do better with home health care than with institutionalization. Home care is desired by more patients and their families because it is wanted by more sick people and their loved ones.

Finding the fallacies in her paper was the first step Carmen needed to take to correct the fallacious arguments she had written.

Directions: Help Carmen find the fallacies in her paper. Label all circular reasoning fallacies with a "CR." Label all jumping to conclusion fallacies with "Jump." Determine the cause and the effect in her cause and effect statements. Mark "C" for cause and "E" for effect. Make sure that the effect logically follows the cause regardless of how the sentence is structured.

▼ APPLYING RECOGNIZING FALLACIES

Carmen feels confident that she has found all the fallacies in her paper. It is now her responsibility to eliminate these fallacies and replace them with more logically constructed arguments. She must also confirm that her cause and effect statements make sense. Following are the strategies Carmen should follow to make her corrections:

Circular Reasoning, or Begging the Question

- Make sure that the conclusion of a statement is not just a restatement of the premise.
- In your argument, do not assume ahead of time that the premise is true.
- Write a conclusion that logically develops from the premise.

Cause and Effect Error

- Write your cause and effect statements carefully.
- Understand that the cause occurs first in time and then the effect. (The rabid dog bit him and then he died.)
- Realize that it is permissible to write the effect first and then describe the cause. (He died when the rabid dog bit him.)
- Be able to identify the cause and the effect in any of your cause and effect statements.
- Check that the cause and effect statement is logically written.

Jumping to Conclusions

- Do not draw a broad conclusion from just a few examples.
- If you must write the outcome of a small sampling of facts, mention that your conclusion is based on a few examples.

Directions: Reread the excerpt from Carmen's home health care paper. In the space provided, help Carmen rewrite her paper by eliminating the fallacies and writing logical arguments. Refer to the preceding strategies for correcting fallacies and checking cause and effect statements.

▼ EVALUATING RECOGNIZING FALLACIES

Directions: While Carmen is grateful for your help in removing the fallacies in her paper and creating logical arguments, she is still concerned that her paper is not corrected properly. You can reassure Carmen that your suggestions for her paper are logical and reasonable by rereading your corrections and answering the following questions in the space provided.

1. Why did you make the corrections that you did? Explain the reasons you used for making three changes in Carmen's paper. Refer to the correction strategies if necessary.

_____

_____

_____

_____

_____

_____

_____

2. What do you feel were the best strategies for recognizing and correcting the fallacies in Carmen's paper? Explain.

_____

_____

_____

_____

_____

_____

_____

_____

CRITICAL READING

Previewing

Preview this selection. Think about what you already know about this topic. In the space provided, write what you still wish to know.

_____

_____

_____

_____

_____

_____

_____

_____

Questioning

Based on your preview, formulate questions that will help you learn what you still wish to know about the topic. Use the space provided.

_____

_____

_____

_____

_____

_____

_____

_____

Reading

Read the selection.

HOME CARE DEPARTMENT ORDERS

Background Information

This department plans with the patient and/or family for the patient's care in the home with outside agency personnel and assists in obtaining necessary medical equipment. The patient makes the choice of a home care agency when one is ordered by the physician. Some hospitals have a home care component within their system. Other home care agencies (Visiting Nurse Associations) are independent and not affiliated with a particular hospital. Discharge planners or home care coordinators have offices in the hospital and help make arrangements to have home care services started when the patient is discharged. Home care can include skilled nursing, home health aide services, physical therapy, occupational therapy, speech therapy, and medical social work. The discharged patient may also need durable medical equipment (DME), such as a hospital bed, oxygen, a walker, or wheelchair. A separate company (a DME company) usually supplies these patient care items and delivers them to the patient's home.

When a patient is being discharged and home care services are being ordered and planned, the case management department may become involved. Case management acts as a patient's advocate in getting the home care services that best suit the patient's needs and coordinates financial coverage through private insurers, Medicare, and so forth.

Doctors' Orders for Home Care

1. Contact home care to plan for discharge next week
2. Home care to arrange with VNS for nursing service twice weekly upon patient discharge
3. Have home care plan with patient's family for discharge in 2 days

SCHEDULING ORDERS

Background Information

Frequently, while the patient is hospitalized, the doctor may write an order to schedule the patient for various types of tests or examinations performed in specialized hospital departments or outside of the hospital.

It is the health unit coordinator's task to notify the department or facility that performs the test or examination and schedule a time convenient to both the involved department and the patient. It is important to record the scheduled time on the patient's kardex form.

Doctors' Orders that Require Scheduling

Below are examples of doctors' orders that require scheduling. These vary greatly among hospitals, according to the services available.

1. Schedule pt in outpatient department for vaginal examination
2. Schedule pt for psychological testing
3. Schedule pt for diabetic classes
4. Schedule pt for hearing evaluation test
5. Schedule in dental clinic for evaluation and care

COMMUNICATION AND IMPLEMENTATION OF HOME CARE ORDERS

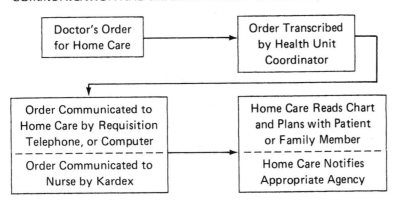

COMMUNICATION AND IMPLEMENTATION OF A DOCTOR'S ORDER THAT REQUIRES SCHEDULING

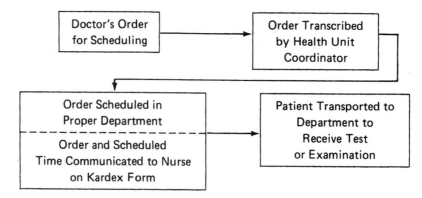

SOCIAL SERVICE DEPARTMENT ORDERS

Background Information

The social service department performs many tasks related to the problems that accompany hospitalization. Money woes, child care worries, obtaining tutors for hospital-bound students, and arranging for transfers to nursing care facilities are some of the problems this department can help solve. Discharge planning may also be coordinated with the home care department to make the transition from the hospital to home easier for the patient.

Doctors' Orders for the Social Services Department

1. Contact husband re: plans to place in nursing facility
2. Arrange for home-bound teacher for 1 month

TEMPORARY ABSENCES (PASSES TO LEAVE THE HOSPITAL)

Some patients may be allowed to leave the hospital for several hours, and other patients who have been confined for a long time may be allowed to leave for several days. Long-term patients receive many benefits from visiting their homes or experiencing a recreational outing. A gradual return to society has therapeutic value for rehabilitating patients.

A temporary pass requires the health unit coordinator to do the following:

1. Arrange with the pharmacy for medications the patient is taking.
2. Note on the census when the patient leaves and returns.

COMMUNICATION AND IMPLEMENTATION OF SOCIAL SERVICE ORDERS

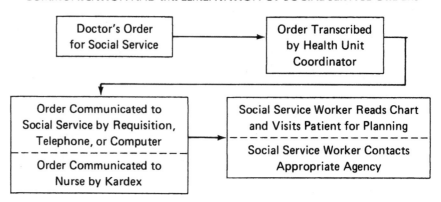

COMMUNICATION AND IMPLEMENTATION OF TEMPORARY ABSENCE ORDERS

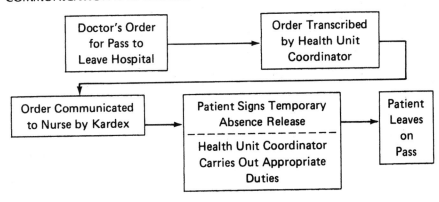

3. Cancel all meals for the length of the absence.
4. Cancel any hospital treatments for the length of the absence.
5. Arrange for any special equipment that the patient may need.
6. Have the patient sign a temporary absence release (Fig. 9–1).

Doctors' Orders for Temporary Absence

1. May have pass for tomorrow from 9 AM to 7 PM
2. Temporary hospital absence from 3 PM Friday to 3 PM Sunday. Arrange for rental of wheelchair.
3. May leave hospital from 10 AM to 1 PM today. Have patient sign permit.

TRANSFER AND DISCHARGE ORDERS

If the doctor plans to transfer the patient to another room or to another unit, or plans to discharge the patient to his or her home or to another facility, he or she writes an order for such on the doctors' order sheet.

To transcribe a transfer or discharge order, the health unit coordinator must notify the hospital admitting department (or discharge department) by telephone, by completing a discharge or transfer slip, or by computer.

Discharge orders may include information, such as instructions for the patient to follow after he or she leaves the hospital, requests for appointments for the patient, and so forth. It is often the task of the health unit coordinator to follow through on completing the order. For example, if the doctor writes "Discharge tomorrow, do not shower for three days," it may be the health unit coordinator's task to write the instructions down on a piece of paper and give it to the patient.

COMMUNICATION AND IMPLEMENTATION OF TRANSFER AND DISCHARGE ORDERS

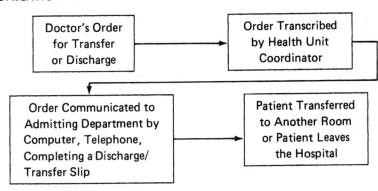

TEMPORARY ABSENCE RELEASE

The undersigned, being a patient of The Above Named Hospital, hereby confirms his (or her) agreement and understanding that neither the hospital, its employees, nor the attending physicians shall be responsible for his (or her) care or condition during any absences of the undersigned from the building or resulting from such absences.

Signed_____
PATIENT / PARENT / GUARDIAN

Date_____

Hour_____

Witness_____

09-0366

TEMPORARY ABSENCE RELEASE

Figure 9–1

Temporary absence release form.

The doctor may request a **transfer** of a patient for various reasons, such as for a different type of room accommodation (ward to private), or for more intense nursing care (regular unit to ICU). Another reason for a transfer is if the patient's condition requires that he or she be placed in an isolation unit.

Later on in the text we will cover the procedures for transferring and discharging a patient. Here we have dealt only with the transcription procedures for a transfer or discharge order.

Doctors' Orders for Transfer or Discharge of a Patient

Below are examples of how discharge or transfer orders may be expressed by the doctor on the doctors' order sheet.

Transfer

1. Transfer patient to 3E please
2. Transfer patient to a private room
3. Transfer patient to ICU after surgery
4. Transfer patient out of ICU to semiprivate room

Discharge

1. Home today
2. Discharge
3. Home $\bar{c}$ R$_x$
4. Home make appt to see me in 2 wk
5. Home $\bar{c}$ crutches

MISCELLANEOUS ORDERS

There are orders that do not relate to any department that are nevertheless deserving of mention. All should be kardexed in their appropriate places. A few of the orders appear below.

1. No visitors or limited number of visitors

A sign should be posted on the patient's door to see the nurse for further explanation. The switchboard and information desk should also be notified.

2. DNR (do not resuscitate) or no code

This order means that no resuscitative measures are to be performed. Some facilities have defined "code-related" categories. An example is "all but CPR." The category of the patient's code status (if one is established) may be required to be indicated on the patient's identification bracelet at the time the admission is being processed. If a code status order is written by the physician, the order should be visible on the kardex and on the patient's chart.

3. NINP (no information, no publication)

Your hospital may use a different abbreviation, but whatever words or abbreviation is used, this order means that the unit denies having the patient and no news concerning the patient is to be given to the press or friends. This order may also be extended to include family members.

4. Notify Dr. Craig of patient's admission to the hospital

This order is not for a consultation. The patient may have been admitted to a surgical service and the surgeon wants the patient's medical doctor to know the patient is in the hospital.

5. Notify HO if systolic pressure above 200

House officer is the name given to the resident on call.

Applying

In the space provided, answer your questions.

_____

_____

_____

_____

_____

_____

_____

Evaluation

Were you able to answer all your questions? Yes _____ No _____

Check the accuracy of your answers by locating the specific information in the selection.

Did the selection give you enough information about the topic? Explain.

_____

_____

_____

_____

_____

_____

_____

STUDENT JOURNAL

List what you have learned about recognizing fallacies	How would you apply this knowledge to your study or work in the health fields?

UNIT III

Applying Critical Thinking Skills to Mathematics

Critical thinking is essential for your success in mathematics. When you are expected to complete mathematical computations in school or at work, you have to follow logical strategies to find accurate solutions.

Problem solving involves *understanding, interpreting, applying,* and *evaluating* mathematical facts. Knowing how to use these critical thinking strategies will improve your abilities in mathematics.

Unit III helps you learn how to apply critical thinking strategies to mathematics. Chapter 10, Using Measurements and Conversions, shows you the different types of measurements and how to convert them from the English system to the metric system. Chapter 11, Comprehending Word Problems, helps you recognize the specific terminology, signals, and processes needed to solve word problems. In Chapter 12, Using Mathematics in the Workplace, you learn how to apply mathematics to work situations.

Unit III will help you learn the specific processes and thinking skills that will improve your abilities in mathematical computations, concepts, and applications in school or at work.

Chapter 10

Using Measurements and Conversions

EXERCISE 10–1

▼ LEARNING OBJECTIVES

In this chapter you will learn how to

- Change terms of measurements from the English system to the metric system.
- Change terms of measurements from the metric system to the English system.
- Do practical conversion problems.

▼ PREDICTING VOCABULARY

Directions: Preview this chapter by finding five words that you recognize but whose precise definition you don't know. Use your background knowledge to write a sentence for each word that predicts the definition of that word.

Word 1: _____

Sentence: _____

_____

Word 2: _____

Sentence: _____

_____

Word 3: _____

Sentence: _____

_____

Word 4: _____

Sentence: _____

_____

Word 5: _____

Sentence: _____

_____

When you finish reading this chapter, evaluate the accuracy of your sentences. Make any necessary revisions.

Revisions

_____

_____

_____

_____

_____

_____

_____

_____

_____

_____

▼ UNDERSTANDING MEASUREMENTS AND CONVERSIONS

After you have had time to survey your new health care textbooks, you will notice that lengths, liquids, weights, and areas are not measured in the manner with which you are familiar. You do not see inches, feet, yards, miles, quarts, ounces, pounds, or tons. Instead you notice such terms for measurement as meter, centimeter, kilometer, millimeter, liter, gram, kilogram, and metric ton. These terms of measurement make up the **metric system** and are used worldwide in the health care professions. Our more common terms of measurement, like inch and pound, are taken from the **English system** and are used in only a few countries, including the United States.

To function successfully in the health care environment, you will need to become proficient in using the metric system. The first strategy for making the transition from the English system to the metric system is to see what English system measurements are equal to what metric system measurements. Table 10–1 will help you visualize the relationship between the English system and the metric system.

TABLE 10–1 Metric System and English System Conversion Chart

Metric Lengths	English Lengths
1 meter =	39.37 inches
1 meter =	3.28 feet
1 meter =	1.09 yards
1 centimeter =	0.4 inch
1 millimeter =	0.04 inch
1 kilometer =	0.62 mile
English Lengths	**Metric Lengths**
1 inch =	25.4 millimeters
1 inch =	2.54 centimeters
1 inch =	0.0254 meter
1 foot =	0.3 meter
1 yard =	0.91 meter
1 mile =	1.61 kilometers
Metric Liquid Measures	**English Liquid Measures**
1 liter =	1.06 quarts
English Liquid Measures	**Metric Liquid Measures**
1 quart =	0.95 liter
Metric Measure of Weight	**English Measure of Weight**
1 gram =	0.04 ounce
1 kilogram =	2.2 pounds
1 metric ton =	2204.62 pounds
English Measure of Weight	**Metric Measure of Weight**
1 ounce =	28.35 grams
1 pound =	0.45 kilogram
1 short ton =	0.91 metric ton
Metric Measure of Area	**English Measure of Area**
1 square centimeter =	0.155 square inch
1 square meter =	10.76 square feet
1 square meter =	1.2 square yards
1 square kilometer =	0.39 square mile
English Measure of Area	**Metric Measure of Area**
1 square inch =	6.45 square centimeters
1 square foot =	0.09 square meter
1 square yard =	0.84 square meter
1 square mile =	2.59 square kilometers

EXERCISE **10-2**

Directions: List some situations in which you have seen the metric system used. Write your answer in the space provided.

_____

_____

_____

_____

_____

_____

EXERCISE **10-3**

Directions: Study Table 10–1. Then determine what metric system terms of measurement could be substituted for the English system terms of measurement listed below. Write your answer in the space next to the English system measurement.

1. mile _____

2. yard _____

3. quart _____

4. short ton _____

5. foot _____

6. ounce _____

7. square mile _____

8. square inch _____

9. pound _____

10. square foot _____

▼ INTERPRETING MEASUREMENTS AND CONVERSIONS

Converting, or changing, from one system of measurement to the other system of measurement is easy if you know how to multiply and have access to a conversion chart like the one above.

The general procedure for changing from the metric system to the English system is to multiply the amount of the metric measure by its equivalent in the English system. For example, to change 6 liters to quarts, multiply 6 by 1.06.

$$6 \times 1.06 = 6.36 \text{ quarts}$$

The general procedure for changing from the English system to the metric system is to multiply the amount of the English measure by its equivalent in the metric system. For example, to change 4 pounds into kilograms, multiply 4 by 0.45 kilogram.

$$4 \times 0.45 = 1.8 \text{ kilograms}$$

Directions: Complete the following statements in the space provided. Refer to the conversion chart above, if necessary.

1. To change pounds to kilograms, multiply the amount in pounds by

   _____.

2. To change kilograms to pounds, multiply the amount in kilograms by

   _____.

3. To change meters to feet, multiply the amount in meters by _____.

4. To change feet to meters, multiply the amount in feet by _____.

5. To change grams to ounces, multiply the amount in grams by _____.

6. To change ounces to grams, multiply the amount in ounces by _____.

7. To change miles to kilometers, multiply the amount in miles by _____.

8. To change kilometers to miles, multiply the amount in kilometers by

   _____.

9. To change square centimeters to square inches, multiply the amount in

   square centimeters by _____.

10. To change square inches to square centimeters, multiply the amount in

    square inches by _____.

Directions: Solve the following conversion problems. Consult the conversion chart, if necessary.

1. Change the following measurements to ounces.

   a. 10 grams _____

   b. 6 grams _____

   c. 3 grams _____

   d. 22 grams _____

   e. 48 grams _____

2. Change the following measurements to square yards.

   a. 12 square meters _____

   b. 32 square meters _____

   c. 59 square meters _____

   d. 87 square meters _____

   e. 105 square meters _____

3. Change the following measurements to inches.

   a. 16 centimeters _____

   b. 29 centimeters _____

   c. 66 centimeters _____

   d. 178 centimeters _____

   e. 321 centimeters _____

4. Change the following measurements to metric tons.

   a. 5 short tons _____

   b. 57 short tons _____

   c. 197 short tons _____

   d. 283 short tons _____

   e. 552 short tons _____

5. Change the following measurements to liters.

   a. 18 quarts _____

   b. 37 quarts _____

   c. 273 quarts _____

   d. 639 quarts _____

   e. 1751 quarts _____

▼ APPLYING MEASUREMENTS AND CONVERSIONS

Whether in your personal life, in your health care workplace, or in your travels abroad, you will need to convert measurements from one system to the other with ease. The following practical problems will provide you with practice in converting the terms of measurement.

Directions: Answer the following word problems in the space provided.

1. What is the weight in ounces of a can of tomatoes that weighs 794 grams?

2. What is the weight in ounces of a can of beans that weighs 454 grams?

3. What is the difference in weight between the can of tomatoes and the can of beans?

4. Car 1 traveled 91 kilometers in one afternoon. Car 2 traveled 60 miles. Which care went farther? How many miles farther did that car go than the other car?

5. The annual rainfall in Montreal is about 970 millimeters. How much is that in inches?

6. The average annual rainfall in Singapore is about 95 inches. How much is that in millimeters?

7. Almost 140,000,000 square miles of the earth is covered by water. How much is that in square kilometers?

8. Mrs. Lima is 159 centimeters tall. Her spouse is 170 centimeters tall. What is the difference, in inches, in their height?

9. Mr. Cipriano's hospital room is 106 meters from the elevator. Approximately how many feet does he have to walk to get to the elevator?

10. Nurse Milton has 10 yards of bandages to fold. How many meters is that?

11. Nurse Clinton has 48 feet of bandages to fold. How many meters is that?

12. Which nurse folded more bandages and by how many meters?

13. For a party for the home health care workers, Marion bought 24 liters of soda pop. Approximately how many quarts of soda pop did he buy?

14. Cassandra is considering a new job as a medical assistant in England. She needs to rent an apartment that will hold all her furniture. Her current American apartment is 800 square feet. How many square meters must her new apartment be to hold all her furniture?

15. How many ounces would 25 grams of baby formula be?

16. Patricia needs to make a hem on her new white uniform dress. She wants to shorten the dress by $3\frac{1}{2}$ inches. How many centimeters is that?

17. Mr. Friedman weighs 98 kilograms. How much does he weigh in pounds?

18. The new CAT scanner weighs $2\frac{1}{2}$ tons. What is the weight in metric tons?

19. The average size of the hospital room is 3 square meters. How large is the room in square feet?

20. Donald was asked to order 18 meters of rubber tubing. How many inches does that represent?

▼ EVALUATING MEASUREMENTS AND CONVERSIONS

To judge if you solved the conversion problems correctly, you can see whether your answers make sense in relation to the numbers given in the problem. For example, if you need to determine how many liters 10 quarts is, you can estimate your answer to be in the range of 10×0.95 liters or 9.5 liters. If your answer was 95 liters, you realize that this total makes no sense for the data given in the problem: 95 liters is much too great a number for a 1 quart = 0.95 liter problem. So when you evaluate whether your conversion answers are correct or not, think in terms of the facts given in the problem.

Directions: Justify the accuracy of each of your solutions in Exercise 10–6. Go over each of the 20 problems. Indicate whether your answers make sense for the numbers given in each problem and the terms of measurements given in the conversion charts. Write your responses in the corresponding spaces below.

Problem Number

1. _____

    _____

2. _____

    _____

3. _____

    _____

4. _____

    _____

5. _____

    _____

6. _____

    _____

7. _____

    _____

8. _____

    _____

9. _____

_____

10. _____

_____

11. _____

_____

12. _____

_____

13. _____

_____

14. _____

_____

15. _____

_____

16. _____

_____

17. _____

_____

18. _____

_____

19. _____

_____

20. _____

_____

CRITICAL READING

Previewing

Preview this selection. Think about what you already know about this topic.
In the space provided, write what you still need to know.

_____

_____

_____

_____

_____

Questioning

Based on your preview, formulate questions that will help you learn what you still wish to know about the topic. Use the space provided.

_____

_____

_____

_____

_____

Reading

Read the following selection from _Health Unit Coordinating_ (LaFleur-Brooks, pp. 184-188).

Component One—Name of the Drug

It is impossible for you to learn the names of all the drugs on the market; therefore, as a beginning or new health unit coordinator you may wish to keep a small notebook with an

COMMUNICATION AND IMPLEMENTATION OF MEDICATION ORDERS

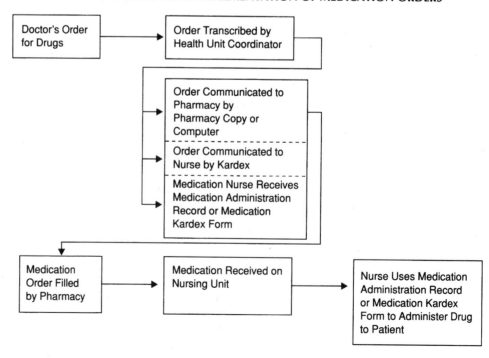

alphabetical index to jot down names of drugs that you encounter frequently. Periodic reviewing will help you to become more familiar with medication names.

Many medications are prepared in different forms, depending on their use (Fig. 10–1). The form is often included with the name of the drug, such as Neosporin *ointment*. For example, ointments are used on the skin or the mucous membranes of the body. Other medications may include a letter as shown in 2 and 3 below.

Examples of Doctors' Medication Orders That Indicate a Specific Form of Medication

1. Neosporin ung ophthalmic OD bid
   Ophthalmic indicates that this ointment is to be used in the eye only.
2. aspirin EC tab ī q3h prn
   The *enteric-coated* (EC) aspirin dissolves only in the small intestine.
3. aspirin T-R 650 mg po q hs
   Time released (T-R) aspirin has a longer lasting effect.
4. aspirin supp 325 mg q3h for temp 101 (R)
   Aspirin is contained in *suppository* (supp) form for insertion into the rectum.

Component Two—Dosage of Drugs

The apothecary system and the metric system are the two methods of weights and measures in present-day hospital use. The **metric system,** which is based on multiples of ten,

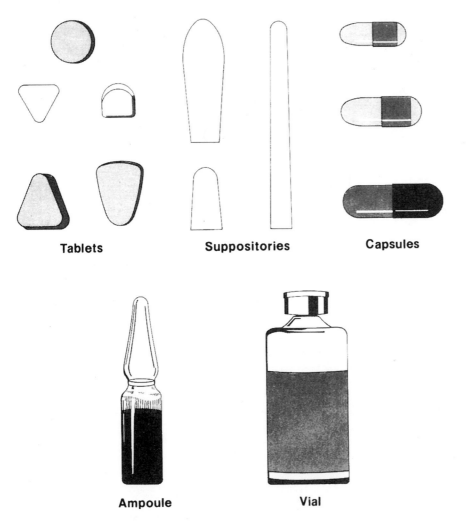

Tablets   **Suppositories**   **Capsules**

Ampoule   **Vial**

Figure 10–1
Common forms of medication.

is the system of choice in scientific fields and is gradually replacing the apothecary system. However, until the apothecary system is completely phased out, the health unit coordinator must continue to be knowledgeable about both systems.

Apothecary System

The **apothecary system** for weighing and measuring drugs and solutions is an ancient system that was brought to the United States from England during the colonial period. Only those terms still used frequently today are listed below.

Terms Relating to Weight (Solid or Powder)
grain (gr)
dram (dr)
ounce (oz)

Terms Relating to Volume (Liquid)
minim (m)
fluid dram (fl dr)
fluid ounce (fl oz)

The abbreviation fl is not always used.

Measurements in this system are written in lowercase Roman numerals. These numerals have a line over them and may be dotted to avoid confusion with similar-appearing letters or numerals. Also the unit of measure precedes the numeral.

Example: one grain—gr ī
five grains—gr v̇

A medication dosage that is less than 1 is written as a fraction.

Example: one sixth grain—gr $\frac{1}{6}$

Remembering that one-half may also be written as s̈s, it is then proper to write one and one-half grains as gr īs̈s and one-half ounce as oz s̈s.

Metric System

The metric system is used everywhere except the United States. The weight, volume, and measurement units are used in other hospital departments as well as in the pharmacy. These basic units are:

Weight = gram (g)
Volume = liter (L)
Length = meter (M)

Smaller and larger units in the metric system can be indicated by attaching prefixes to the basic units. This text will not cover all the prefixes used in the metric system because not all are used in doctors' orders.

To enlarge the basic unit 1000 times, the prefix *kilo* is added.

Example: kilogram (kg) = 1000 g

To diminish the basic unit by 100, the prefix *centi* is added. The prefix *milli* diminishes the basic unit by 1000. A milligram (mg), milliliter (mL), millimeter (mm) represent 1/1000 of the basic unit. The symbol μ represents the prefix *micro*.

Example: 1 μm = 1 micrometer or 0.001 millimeter

The terms *milliliter* (mL) and *cubic centimeter* (cc) are used interchangeably, although milliliter is preferred.

Example: 1 L = 1000 cc or 1000 mL

The metric system uses the Arabic numerals that we all know—1, 2, 3, and so forth. Abbreviations are placed after the number, as in 50 mg or 500 mL.

Quantities less than 1 and fractions are written in decimal form, for example: 0.25 mg, 1.25 mg, 1.5 g.

Abbreviations used in medication dosages that *do not fall* within the apothecary or metric systems are: gtt (drop), mEq (milliequivalent), and U (unit). Examples of their usage in doctors' orders are:

pilocarpine 1% gtts ii OU tid
add 40 mEq KCl to each IV
Bicillin 600,000 U bid × 3 days

Table 10–2 lists approximate equivalents between the two systems. There are times when knowledge of the equivalents will prove helpful to the health unit coordinator.

Component Three—Routes of Administration

Medications may be administered to patients using different routes of administration. Also, any one medication may be prepared to be given by several different methods. Doctors should always indicate the route of administration. However, when a medication can be given only by mouth, the route is frequently omitted in the doctor's order. The following list contains the routes most frequently used in medication administration, with an example of each.

1. *Oral (mouth or po)*
   The patient swallows the medication, which may be in the form of a capsule, pill, tablet, spansule, or liquid.
   Example: Librium 10 mg po tid

2. *Sublingual*
   The tablet is placed under the tongue, where it is absorbed.
   Example: nitroglycerin gr 1/150 subling prn anginal pain

3. *Inhalation*
   These liquid medications are most commonly administered by the respiratory care department as part of their treatment procedure.

4. *Topical*
   Applied to skin or mucous membrane. Medications in this category may be in the form of lotions, liniments, ointments, powders, sprays, solutions, suppositories, or transderm preparations.

TABLE 10–2   Approximate Equivalent Weights and Volume for Metric and Apothecary Systems

Metric	Apothecary
Weight	
60 or 65 mg	gr ī
100 mg	gr īss
300 or 325 mg	gr v̄
500 mg or 0.5 g	gr v̄īīss
0.4 mg	gr 1/150
15 mg	gr 1/4
10 mg	gr 1/6
32 mg	gr ss
Volume	
30 cc or 30 mL (mL and cc interchangeable)	fl oz ī
500 cc or 0.5 L	fl oz x̄v̄ī (pt)
1000 cc or 1 L	fl oz x̄x̄xīī (qt)

a. Applied to the skin.

Example 1: apply Neosporin ointment to rt leg ulcer bid.

Example 2: Transderm-Nitro 5 ī qd. (The medication is part of a flat disk that is applied to the body, usually the chest; the medication is released over a specified period.)

b. Spraying onto skin or mucous membrane

Example 1: spray lt ankle wound with Neosporin aerosol tid

Example 2: Chloraseptic throat spray q3h prn for throat irritation

c. Instillation

These liquids are dropped into the eye, ear, or nose.

Examples: Eye—Neosporin ophth sol'n gtts ī̄ī OS bid.

Ear—Cortisporin otic suspension gtts ī̄īī in lt ear qid

Nose—Neo-Synephrine 0.5% nose drops ī̄ī in each nostril q4h prn nasal congestion

d. Insertions of drugs into body openings—suppositories

1. Rectal

Example: Compazine supp 5 mg q4h prn N/V

2. Vaginal

Example: Mycostatin vag supp ī. Insert each AM

5. Parenteral

Fluids or medications given by injection or intravenously.

a. Intradermal

Injected between two skin layers. These injections are principally for diagnostic testing.

Example: PPD intermediate today. PPD (purified protein derivative) is a tuberculin skin test order. The word "intermediate" indicates the strength of the drug.

b. Subcutaneous (SC)

The medication is injected with a syringe under the skin into the fat or connective tissue.

Example: heparin 5000 U SC stat

c. Intramuscular (IM)

The medication is injected directly into the muscle.

Example: Demerol 50 mg IM stat

d. Intravenous

The medication is injected within the vein.

i. IV push or bolus—A concentrated amount of medication given within a vein.

Example: Lanoxin 0.125 mg IV push (slowly) stat

ii. Intravenous piggyback (IVPB)—The medication added to a small amount of commercially prepared IV solution (50–100 mL) and infused through an established IV line (Fig. 10–2).

Example: Keflin 0.5 g IVPB q6h

iii. Admixture—Adding one or more medications to a commercially prepared intravenous solution. It is usually prepared by the pharmacy. The medication(s) are infused by vein all during the time the IV is running.

Example: 1000 cc 5% D/W to run at 125 cc/h. Add 20 mEq KCl.

iv. Heparin lock—This device is used for administering intermittent IV therapy infusions when continuous IV solutions are not necessary. It is also used to keep a vein "open" for emergency medications.

6. Intravenous Hyperalimentation or Total Parenteral Nutrition

Sometimes, because of the nature of the illness, the patient is not able to take in orally all of the necessary nutrients and calories needed by the body. The conventional intravenous solutions cannot provide the protein and calories required; therefore, total parenteral nutrition (TPN) or IV hyperalimentation is ordered. The term *partial parenteral nutrition* (PPN) refers to the intravenous provision of partial nutritional requirements.

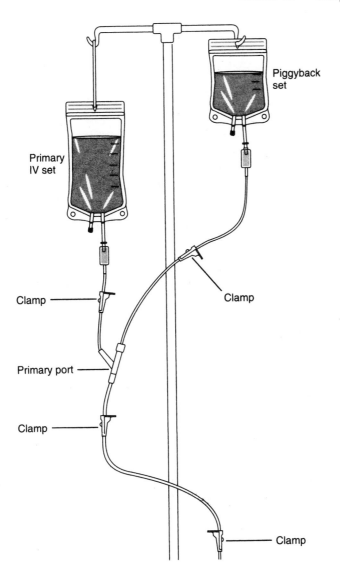

Figure 10–2
An intravenous set with piggyback bags.

Piggyback set

Primary IV set

Clamp

Clamp

Primary port

Clamp

Clamp

The central venous catheter through which the feeding is given is inserted under sterile conditions by the doctor. These types of catheters not only deliver nutrition to the patient but they have other uses, such as a means of collecting blood specimens from patients without repeated venipunctures. The most common types of central venous catheters are the Hickman or Broviac catheter, the Groshong catheter and the implanted venous access ports, such as Med-I-Port, Infus-A-Port, Port-A-Cath. These catheters are similar to each other but each has special features making their use appropriate for certain applications. An infusion pump controls the rate at which the TPN is delivered. The TPN solution should be kept refrigerated until ready to use.

Infection is a possible risk to patients receiving TPN and therefore their temperatures are taken more frequently. There is also the possibility of glucose intolerance; therefore, urine reductions are usually ordered every 6 h.

A consent form is needed for implanting a central venous catheter. A form for ordering the feeding is shown in Figure 10–3.

The order for these IV feedings, which may be administered to babies as well as to children and adults, is of some length, as you will see in the example below. The regular transcription procedure is followed.

PID

ADULT TOTAL PARENTERAL NUTRITION (TPN) ORDER

An adult TPN Order Form must be sent to the Pharmacy
EVERY DAY by noon and always include the infusion rate. The total
volume prepared for a 24 hour supply is calculated from the infusion
rate.

Each liter of Standard Balanced TPN contains approx. 1000 calories to
be administered by CENTRAL LINE ONLY.

Any variations to the Standard Balanced TPN must be written on the
ADULT TPN Order form. Any change in electrolyte content must include
both cation and anion.

DATE:	INFUSION RATE:		☒ Check this box to order STANDARD BALANCED TPN.	
	_____ ml/hr.			

ADDITIVES PER 1000 ml.	1000ml: Standard Balanced TPN contains:	ENTER CHANGES TO STANDARD BALANCED TPN BELOW:
PROTEIN: AMINO ACIDS	42.5 Gms	
CARBOHYDRATE: DEXTROSE	250.0 Gms	
ELECTROLYTES: SODIUM ION	49. mEq	
POTASSIUM ION	40. mEq	
MAGNESIUM ION	8. mEq	
CALCIUM ION	10. mEq	
CHLORIDE ION	49. mEq	
PHOSPHATE ION	22. mEq	
ACETATE ION	92. mEq	
VITAMINS: MVI CONCENTRATE TO 1ST BOTTLE	5. ml	
TRACE ELEMENTS: ZINC SULFATE	5. mg	
COPPER SULFATE	1.mg	
OTHER:		

SPECIAL
INSTRUCTIONS: _____

_____

_____

10% FAT EMULSIONS 500 ml.   ☐ NO   ☐ YES   IF YES, _____ ml./hr.

081 3001 10-81

CHART COPY (White)
PHARMACY COPY (Yellow)   _____
                          (Physician's Signature)

Figure 10–3

Total parenteral nutrition order form.

Applying

In the space provided, answer your questions.

_____

_____

_____

_____

_____

_____

_____

Evaluating

Were you able to answer all your questions? Yes _____ No _____

Check the accuracy of your answers by locating the specific information in the selection.

Did the selection give you enough information about the topic? Explain.

_____

_____

_____

_____

_____

_____

_____

STUDENT JOURNAL

List what you have learned about measurements and conversions.	How would you apply this knowledge to your study or work in the health fields?

Chapter 11

Comprehending
Word Problems

▼ LEARNING OBJECTIVES

In this chapter you learn how to
- Recognize specific terminology and signals needed to solve word problems
- Recognize the processes needed to solve word problems

▼ PREDICTING VOCABULARY

Directions: Preview this chapter by finding five words that you recognize but whose precise definition you don't know. Use your background knowledge to write a sentence for each word that predicts the definition of that word.

Word 1: _____

Sentence: _____

_____

Word 2: _____

Sentence: _____

_____

Word 3: _____

Sentence: _____

_____

Word 4: _____

Sentence: _____

_____

Word 5: _____

Sentence: _____

_____

When you finish reading this chapter, evaluate the accuracy of your sentences. Make any necessary revisions.

Revisions

_____

_____

_____

_____

_____

_____

_____

_____

_____

▼ UNDERSTANDING COMPREHENDING WORD PROBLEMS

Many students become intimidated when they are asked to solve word problems in mathematics. They don't know where to begin. Solving a word problem begins with attacking the problem step by step.

The first step is to write down the information you need to solve the problem. Make sure that you understand the terminology. Write any key mathematical terms and definitions on your paper. Some examples of key terms are _estimate, average, calculate, equation,_ and _deduct._ You cannot solve the problem if you do not know the meanings of the math vocabulary that is used.

The next step is to write down the mathematical process you need to do to solve the problem. Are you asked to _add, subtract, multiply,_ or _divide_ or any combination of these procedures? To check that you have chosen the correct process, write the signal word that identifies that process. For example, the word _total_ signals the process _addition._

Then write the number of steps that are required to solve the word problem. For example, do you have to _add_ (one step) or do you have to first _add_ and then _multiply_ (two steps)?

Writing the information in word problems helps you think about the process necessary to solve the problem.

Example 11–1

Read the following word problem and write the information that you need to find the solution.

John traveled 30 miles on Monday and 40 miles on Tuesday. What was his total mileage? What was his average mileage?

1. The word *average* means a middle point between extremes.
2. The word *total* signals the process addition. The word *average* signals the process division. Therefore, two steps are necessary to solve the problem.
   Step 1: 40 + 30 = 70 total miles
   Step 2: 70/2 = 35 miles per day (average mileage)

Directions: Solve the following word problems by writing the information needed for the solution.

EXERCISE 11-2

1. Monica spent $5.50 for candy bars. Each bar cost $0.25. Calculate the number of candy bars that Monica bought.

   a. The mathematical term *calculate* means _____

   b. The signal word is _____

   c. The process is _____

   d. The number of steps is _____

   e. The answer is _____

2. Maria walked 15 miles to school. She walked 5 miles to work when school was over. Calculate the total number of miles that Maria walked.

   a. The mathematical term *calculate* means _____

   b. The signal word is _____

   c. The process is _____

   d. The number of steps is _____

   e. The answer is _____

3. David got 33 hits out of 99 times at bat. Nancy got 25 hits out of 75 times at bat. Who had the better batting average?

   a. The mathematical term *average* means _____

   b. The signal word is _____

   c. The process is _____

   d. The number of steps is _____

   e. The answer is _____

4. Arthur worked 3.5 hours on Monday and 2.5 hours on Tuesday. He was paid a total of $120.00. Estimate his hourly wage.

   a. The mathematical term *estimate* means _____

   b. The signal word is _____

c. The process is _____

d. The number of steps is _____

e. The answer is _____

5. Don and Mario purchased supplies for a total of $450.75. Don paid $350.80. Deduct Don's payment from the total cost. How much did Mario have to pay?

a. The mathematical term *deduct* means _____

b. The signal word is _____

c. The process is _____

d. The number of steps is _____

e. The answer is _____

▼ INTERPRETING COMPREHENDING WORD PROBLEMS

Interpreting word problems involves closely examining the information in the problem to understand it better. Comparing, contrasting, classifying, or breaking down the facts in the problem will help you find the solution. To interpret word problems, you have to be able to state *why* the facts are needed to solve the problem.

Example 11–2

Read the following word problem and the explanation of why certain facts were needed to solve the problem.

> One computer store listed a software program at $250. A discount store 3 miles away charged $215.99 for the same program. How much can be saved by buying the program at the discount store?

COMPUTER STORE CHARGED $250
DISCOUNT STORE CHARGED $215.99

These details are the only facts needed to solve the problem because the answer is the difference between these two prices.

$250.00
−$215.99
─────────
$34.01   THE ANSWER

Directions: Read the following word problems. Write the facts needed to solve the problems and *why* this information is necessary. Then solve the problem.

1. The total calories in 10 servings of minestrone soup is 175. The total calories in 6 servings of vegetable soup is 180. Which soup has more calories per serving?

a. Facts needed _____

_____

b. Reasons why _____

_____

c. Solution _____

2. Joan and Marian met for dinner at their favorite restaurant. Joan ordered a half order of pasta, which cost $6.95 per order. Marian ordered a Caesar salad for $3.95. Who paid more for dinner?

a. Facts needed _____

_____

b. Reasons why _____

_____

c. Solution _____

3. A fish sandwich at one fast-food restaurant is 425 calories. A competitive restaurant chain offers a fish sandwich at 450 calories. What is the percent difference in the calories?

a. Facts needed _____

_____

b. Reasons why _____

_____

c. Solution _____

4. George runs $2\frac{1}{2}$ miles in the morning before work. After work he runs another $3\frac{1}{4}$ miles. How many miles does he run each day?

a. Facts needed _____

_____

b. Reasons why _____

_____

c. Solution _____

5. A television costs $250. A VCR costs an additional $219. A combined TV-VCR costs $438. Is the combination a better value?

a. Facts needed _____

_____

b. Reasons why _____

_____

c. Solution _____

▼ APPLYING COMPREHENDING WORD PROBLEMS

When you apply the information from word problems, you use the information you've gained from solving the problem. Among the ways you can use this information are to organize facts needed and to apply the facts to make something work. When you apply solutions to problems, you select facts, organize details, and demonstrate how this information is useful.

Example 11–3

Read the information in the word problem and the explanation of how this information can be used.

Examine the following AM train schedule. During which hour do the trains run most often and what is the time between trains?

Train Schedule AM

7:00	9:00
7:40	10:00
8:20	11:00
8:40	12:00

The trains run most frequently between 8:00 and 9:00. The time interval is every 20 minutes. The information is useful if you need to catch a morning train.

Exercise 11–4

Directions: Solve the following word problems. Then explain how you could use the information gained from solving the problem.

1. Sonia lives in New York City and wants to visit her grandmother, who lives 90 miles away. She has to observe a speed limit of 40 miles an hour. How long will it take her to travel to her grandmother's house?

   _____

   _____

   _____

2. Tony weighs 175 pounds. His doctor told him to lose 5 pounds a week for the next 3 weeks. How many pounds does Tony have to lose?

   _____

   _____

   _____

3. Employees A and B were trying to demonstrate efficiency at work. Which employee completed more work (see illustration, p. 191)?

   _____

   _____

   _____

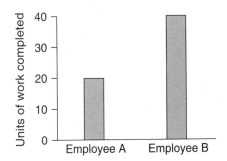

4. Cucumber yogurt dressing is 22 calories per 1³/₄-ounce serving. Honey mustard dressing is 54 calories per 2-ounce serving. Which dressing has fewer calories?

_____

_____

_____

5. John scored the following grades on his tests: 72, 85, 78, and 93. What is his average for the semester?

_____

_____

_____

▼ EVALUATING COMPREHENDING WORD PROBLEMS

When you evaluate your answers to word problems, you judge the accuracy or value of your answer. Evaluation gives you a chance to think about your solution and to explain why your answer makes sense.

Example 11–4

Read the following word problem, its solution, and the explanation of why the answer makes sense.

Frances is 4 feet 7 inches tall. Her sister, Jenny, is 5 feet 3 inches tall. How much taller is Jenny than Frances?

5 feet × 12 inches = 60 + 3 = 63 (Total 1)

4 feet × 12 inches = 48 + 7 = 55 (Total 2)

63 − 55 = 8 inches

The problem was solved by converting feet to inches, adding the total number of inches for each girl, and subtracting total 2 from total 1 to arrive at the answer. The answer, 8 inches, makes sense when you visualize the difference between 55 inches and 63 inches.

EXERCISE
11–5

Directions: Solve the following word problems. Then explain why your answer makes sense.

1. Harvey bought 35 ounces of cheese. Since there are 16 ounces to a pound, approximately how many pounds of cheese did he buy?

_____

_____

_____

_____

2. Mindy baked cookies for the firm's annual picnic. One third of the 2 dozen cookies were chocolate chip. The rest were peanut butter. How many peanut butter cookies did Mindy bake?

_____

_____

_____

_____

3. Michael swam for $3/4$ hour at the rate $2\frac{1}{2}$ miles per hour. How far did he swim?

_____

_____

_____

_____

4. Robert bought a hamburger on a bun for dinner. The ratio of meat to bun was 4:1. The total weight of meat and bun was 8 ounces. What was the weight of the hamburger?

_____

_____

_____

_____

5. Marcy bought a dress and sweater. The dress cost twice as much as the sweater. The sweater cost $35. How much was the dress?

_____

_____

_____

_____

CRITICAL READING

Previewing

Preview this selection. Think about what you already know about this topic. In the space provided, write what you still wish to know.

_____

_____

_____

_____

_____

Questioning

Based on your preview, formulate questions that will help you learn what you still wish to know about the topic.

_____

_____

_____

_____

_____

Reading

Read the following selection from _EMT Prehospital Care_ (Henry and Stapleton, pp. 647-649).

Respiratory Function

The respiratory rate in children is much faster than in the adult, and it gradually decreases with age. Newborns have a respiratory rate of above 40. Infants (up to 1 year) have an average respiratory rate of 24 to 30 breaths/minute, younger children have a rate of 20 to 25 breaths/minute, and older children have a rate of 15 to 20 breaths/minute. You should be generally familiar with the range of variations in order to evaluate the patient's respiratory status properly.

As with the adult, the rate of breathing alone is not the measure of adequate ventilation. Depth of breathing or tidal volume must also be considered. The evaluation of depth is done by observing for chest rise and listening and feeling for the movement of air. When positive-pressure ventilation is necessary, care must be taken not to overventilate, since the respiratory volumes of infants and children also vary with age. During ventilation you must be careful to observe chest rise closely to determine the end-point of ventilation. Infants and small children are more subject to gastric distention because of their small lung capacity and the tendency for excessive volumes and pressure of air to "overflow" into the esophagus.

Infants have very compliant chest walls. When they work harder at breathing and use their accessory muscles of respiration, supraclavicular, substernal, and intercostal retractions are noted along the supple chest wall. Retractions and nasal flaring, which are signs of increased work of breathing, are obvious on inspection. Infants and children can mount a vigorous respiratory and cardiovascular response to compensate for illness. However, since their energy stores are less, children can quite easily decompensate because any significant pathophysiology rapidly tires the muscles of respiration.

Respiratory Effort and Fatigue

When they need to work to breathe, infants and children experience respiratory muscle fatigue more rapidly than adults. When this occurs they may experience a sudden *deterioration* (downhill course) in their condition. For example, children with asthma may be at home for extended periods while the parents attempt to break the attack and avoid hospitalization. During this time, the children experience increased work at breathing and may be unable to sleep. They become exhausted. The EMT must remember that the child may tire to the point where respiratory efforts are inadequate and assistance via positive-pressure ventilation is necessary. Beware when the child who has been working to breathe becomes tired and wants to sleep or lie down. Also, remember that anxiety and anxious behavior may be a sign of hypoxia, which appears before the patient becomes cyanotic.

Simple interventions such as administering high-concentration humidified oxygen and keeping the infant warm extend the *compensatory* or grace period. By adding oxygen you may decrease the need to work so hard at breathing. Except during the newborn period, there is absolutely no contraindication to using high-concentration oxygen. Oxygen toxicity is not a consideration in prehospital transport. Humidifying the oxygen is important, since dried secretions might obstruct airflow and increase airway resistance. Therefore, give humidified oxygen when possible.

Pulse Rate and Blood Pressure

The average pulse rate of the child decreases with age. For example, an infant's average pulse rate is 130 with a range from 100 to 190. Thereafter the average values decrease toward adult values. When evaluating traumatized infants and children, you must be able to appreciate these values in determining the extent of blood loss and the severity of shock.

The blood pressure increases with age. Use the cuff size appropriate for an infant or child to prevent false readings. As a general rule, the width of the cuff should cover approximately two thirds of the length of the upper arm, and the bladder should cover approximately 75% of the arm's circumference. If the cuff is too small, readings are falsely high, and if it is too large, readings are falsely low.

With the greater range and variability in normal vital signs, it is sometimes more difficult to interpret the significance of changes in blood pressure in the child. The American College of Surgeons considers a systolic blood pressure of less than 70 mm Hg with tachycardia and cool skin an indicator of shock in children.

Metabolic Considerations

Keeping the child warm is a simple and valuable measure that should not be underestimated. Infants and children have a higher baseline metabolic rate than adults. Their engine (so to speak) runs at higher rpms. This means that for their size, they need more fuel, which in humans is oxygen and glucose. To accomplish this they have a faster normal respiratory rate to capture the oxygen and a faster normal heart rate to deliver it to the tissues. They also consume more calories per unit weight than do adults, as any bleary-eyed new parent can attest to after nighttime feedings.

Part of the reason infants have a higher basal metabolic rate is that they are busy growing. Another explanation is that they need to expend more energy to remain warm. Notice that infants have proportionately larger heads and a greater skin surface area relative to body weight than do adults. This means they lose heat and moisture through the skin more easily. Their higher respiratory rate also adds to the amount of heat and water lost through the lungs.

The intake of food and water usually decreases in the sick or injured child. This can exhaust the *glycogen* (stored form of glucose) supply during the course of the illness. Since the metabolic rate is higher and because there are smaller reserves of glucose, children quickly use up their energy supplies. Fever will further increase the metabolic rate and complicate this situation.

It is important to keep the sick infant warm; otherwise the infant may consume his or her energy stores just to stay warm. The glycogen stored in the liver is then rapidly depleted and unavailable for other metabolic needs. *Remember, when the metabolic needs on a cellular level are not met, shock results.* A further problem is that infants less than 6 months of age cannot shiver in response to cold and therefore cannot generate heat through muscular contraction. By keeping the child warm and well-oxygenated, you help the infant conserve his or her energy reserves.

Neurologic Differences

The very young pediatric patient's head is large in relation to the body. Thus, this patient is more likely to suffer head injury. The infant is capable of suffering blood loss within the cranium sufficient to cause shock. This is in contrast to the adult and child patient, in whom significant blood loss and hypovolemic shock are not possible with closed head injuries. Both infants and children are also more prone to *apneic* (absence of breathing) episodes with head trauma.

It is important to remember that the infant and child have a greater chance of recovering from brain hypoxia or head trauma than does an adult suffering a similar insult.

Response to Hypovolemia and Shock States

Hypovolemic shock is the most common type of shock in childhood. Acute dehydration and hemorrhage are the two causes of hypovolemia most often encountered by EMTs.

Hypovolemia from *dehydration* (not enough water) is likely in any sick child with increased metabolic needs and poor intake. Vomiting and diarrhea hasten fluid loss. The smaller the child, the more vulnerable that child is to dehydration.

The child tolerates a gradual loss of fluids during acute illness because fluid shifts from the cells and interstitial fluid to maintain the plasma volume. As this occurs, there is a progression of *signs of dehydration*. Initially, the small child or infant has tachycardia, less urine output, and dry mucosal membranes. This progresses to lack of tears, a sunken fontanelle, and sunken eyes. Late signs are skin tenting, delayed capillary refill, hyperventilation, an altered mental status (which includes irritability and lethargy), and a thready pulse. Hypotension is a very late sign.

With acute blood or fluid loss, as occurs in hemorrhage, the pediatric patient exhibits the same signs of shock as an adult. Remember that the total blood volume of children is significantly less than in adults. The average blood volume is 80 ml/kg. This means an average 10-kg 1-year-old infant would have 800 ml of total blood volume. What might be an insignificant 200-ml blood loss in an adult is 25% of the 10-kg baby's blood volume.

With health compensatory mechanisms, children can maintain their blood pressure until nearly 40% of the blood volume is lost. The drop in blood pressure in the child is even a later finding than in adults. By the time children are hypotensive they are in deep shock.

Children and infants are also susceptible to other less common causes of shock. Distributive shock is seen with sepsis, anaphylaxis, and spinal cord shock, as well as in response to certain drugs. Following trauma, the pediatric patient can suffer obstructive shock from tension pneumothorax and cardiac tamponade. Rarely will a child suffer cardiogenic shock. Possible causes of cardiogenic shock in a child include a myocardial contusion, previous congenital heart disease, or an acute *cardiomyopathy* (infection of the myocardium).

Applying

In the space provided, answer your questions.

_____

_____

_____

_____

_____

_____

_____

Evaluating

Were you able to answer all your questions? Yes _____ No _____. Did the selection give you enough information about the topic? Explain.

_____

_____

_____

_____

_____

_____

_____

Check the accuracy of your answers by finding the specific information in the selection.

STUDENT JOURNAL

List what you have learned about comprehending word problems.	How would you apply this knowledge to your study or work in the health fields?

Chapter 12

Using Mathematics in the Workplace

▼ **LEARNING OBJECTIVES**

In this chapter you learn how to
• Apply mathematics to work situations

▼ **PREDICTING VOCABULARY**

Directions: Preview this chapter by finding five words that you recognize but whose precise definition you don't know. Use your background knowledge to write a sentence for each word that predicts the definition of that word.

Word 1: _____

Sentence: _____

_____

Word 2: _____

Sentence: _____

_____

Word 3: _____

Sentence: _____

_____

Word 4: _____

Sentence: _____

_____

Word 5: _____

Sentence: _____

_____

When you finish reading this chapter, evaluate the accuracy of your sentences. Make any necessary revisions.

Revisions

_____

_____

_____

_____

_____

_____

_____

_____

▼ UNDERSTANDING USING MATHEMATICS IN THE WORKPLACE

Many workers become confused when they have to use mathematics in the workplace. They may make errors and have employment problems because they have not learned how to apply basic math skills to on-the-job situations. For example, workers have to know when it's appropriate to make estimations and when exact numbers are required.

The employment situation may require workers to use numbers to measure and record temperature, prepare budgets, count calories or fat content for diets, or use metric measurements. Knowing how to use math skills is a necessity in a number of workplace situations.

The first step is to make sure that you know your basic math skills. The next step is to know how to use your math skills to do your work correctly. You have to understand which specific skills to apply to the tasks required on the job.

Example 12-1

Joan was required to order a low-calorie breakfast menu for a patient. She looked at a chart that listed the calories of certain foods. To do this job task successfully, she had to *add* the *total* number of calories. She determined that it was necessary to use the skill *addition* to fulfill this assignment at work.

Item	Calories
Oatmeal	145
Coffee	4
Skim milk	80
Fruit	130
TOTAL	359

EXERCISE
12–2

Directions: Read each workplace task. Determine which math skill (addition, subtraction, multiplication, division) or combination of math skills should be used to complete the job task. Then complete each math problem.

1. Erica is required to complete the payment schedule for employees in the medical office. She notices that Dan was absent 4 days. His monthly check for 20 days of work each month is $1750. How much should she deduct from Dan's monthly pay check?

   Math Skill _____

   Answer _____

2. Harold had to purchase 12 pounds of apples. The apples cost 98 cents per pound. What was the total cost of Harold's purchase?

   Math Skill _____

   Answer _____

3. Judy had a bookshelf built in her office. The height of her office from floor to ceiling was 4 meters. She wanted to have 12 rows of shelves installed. Calculate the height of each shelf in centimeters.

   Math Skill _____

   Answer _____

4. Melinda's office in New York needed equipment shipped from California. Melinda was asked to order the equipment by phone at 4 PM Pacific Standard Time. Eastern Standard Time is 3 hours ahead. What time is it in New York?

   Math Skill _____

   Answer _____

5. Juan placed an order for computer software. The company promised delivery in 2 weeks. The software arrived 23 days after he placed the order. How late was the delivery?

   Math Skill _____

   Answer _____

▼ INTERPRETING USING MATHEMATICS IN THE WORKPLACE

Using mathematics in the workplace often involves looking closely at the numerical facts to complete a job task. Sometimes workers are asked to compare numbers or combine numerical facts to do their jobs. At other times workers have to choose the correct numerical facts or organize mathematical information to perform their work tasks.

Example 12–2

A patient was complaining about side effects of his medication. Todd decided to look at the patient's chart to check information about the patient's medicine. Todd checked the prescribed dosage on the chart. The patient was taking twice the dosage indicated on the chart. Todd alerted the physician, and the patient was then given careful instructions about the proper dosage. Todd did two correct procedures. First he checked the numerical facts on the chart. Then he compared those numbers to the actual number of doses taken by the patient and realized the discrepancy. Therefore he alerted the doctor to give the patient the correct information. A close look at numerical facts saved this patient from medical complications.

Directions: Read each workplace situation. Decide which mathematical facts are necessary to get the job done. Put a check next to the facts needed to solve the problem. Then solve the problem.

EXERCISE **12–3**

1. Milk costs $2.00 per gallon. Mike had to purchase 4 quarts of milk for the hospital cafeteria. What was the total cost?

   Which fact(s) are needed?
   a. 4 quarts are in a gallon
   b. 40 quarts = 10 gallons
   c. $2.00 is a high price for milk

   Answer _____

2. Sandy was trying to determine the fat content in the dinner menu. One ounce of American cheese has 77% fat calories. One ounce of Swiss cheese has 67% fat. What is the fat percentage saved by eating Swiss cheese instead of American cheese?

   Which fact(s) are needed?
   a. 1 ounce of American cheese has 77% fat calories
   b. 1 ounce of Swiss cheese has 67% fat calories
   c. Sandy was eating cheese for dinner

   Answer _____

3. A person needs 2.5 L of water each day to survive. John is going on a hike. Now much water does he need for 3 days?

   Which fact(s) are needed?
   a. John is going on a hike
   b. A person needs 2.5 L of water each day
   c. He needs water for 3 days

   Answer _____

4. What percentage of the health care center's budget is spent on salaries?

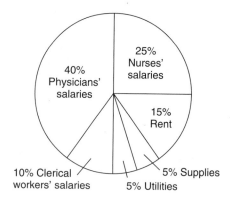

Budget For Health Care Center

Which fact(s) are needed?
a. Physicians' salaries 40%
b. Nurses' salaries 25%
c. Clerical workers' salaries 10%

Answer _____

5. The driver of the EMS vehicle can travel 28 km in 20 minutes. How long will it take the driver to travel 56 km?

Which fact(s) are needed?
a. The driver is driving an EMS vehicle
b. The driver travels 28 km in 20 minutes
c. The total distance will be 56 km

Answer _____

▼ APPLYING USING MATHEMATICS IN THE WORKPLACE

When you have to apply mathematics to the workplace, several tasks are involved. First, you have to identify the essential information required to fulfill the job task. Then you are required to organize that information. You have to interpret the mathematical facts and use those facts to complete a work assignment successfully.

Example 12–3

Read the following example and explanation of the application to the job task.

Larry is required to measure one wall of his office so that it can be wood paneled. The wall is 9 meters wide and 4 meters high. The wood paneling costs $10 a square meter. How much will it cost to panel the wall? Make a plan for Larry's paneling job.

Larry first has to measure the wall. Then he has to multiply $10 times the total number of square meters. Once he has the total cost, he can order the panels and complete the job.

Directions: Read the following mathematical problems. Use the mathematical facts to complete the assigned job tasks.

1. There are 30 employees in the office. The office has supplied 160 packages of Xerox paper as the supply for the year. How can you, as the office manager, distribute this supply so that the paper will last a year?

_____

_____

_____

2. The exterior of your office building has to be cleaned. The building is 1000 feet high and 300 feet wide. One cleaning service bid $0.30 a square foot. Another service bid $0.25 a square foot. How much money will you save by using the second service?

_____

_____

_____

3. A temporary worker earns $6.00 per hour. A full-time employee earns $8.50 per hour plus another $1.50 per hour for benefits. How much money can you save in one 40-hour week by replacing two full-time employees with two temporary workers?

_____

_____

_____

4. You are looking for medical office space 0.3 km from the nearest hospital. The space you found was 0.8 km from the hospital. How much farther is it from the hospital than the space you desired?

_____

_____

_____

5. You are responsible for the training program of 75 home health care workers. Forty of these workers passed the training program. What percentage of the training class will have to repeat the course?

_____

_____

_____

▼ EVALUATING USING MATHEMATICS IN THE WORKPLACE

Once you've completed your job task, you have to judge whether you correctly used the numerical facts at hand to fulfill your assignment.

Example 12–4

Read the following description of Alice's job task and her evaluation of her ability to use the given mathematical facts to complete the assignment successfully.

Alice has to fit six dental appointments into Dr. Meade's Thursday afternoon schedule. Dr. Meade's hours on Thursday afternoon are from 1 to 5. One appointment will take at least an hour. The rest are routine checkups. How should Alice set up Dr. Meade's Thursday afternoon schedule?

1st appointment	1:00-2:00
2nd appointment	2:05-2:35
3rd appointment	2:40-3:10
4th appointment	3:15-3:45
5th appointment	3:55-4:25
6th appointment	4:30-5:00

Alice decided to schedule the longest appointment first so that Dr. Meade could begin with his most difficult case. Then she divided the remaining appoints by converting hours into minutes and dividing by 5. She had time to schedule 5-minute breaks between patients and still finish Dr. Meade's day by 5 PM. Alice fulfilled her job task because she understood what her work assignment was and she recognized the mathematical facts she needed to complete her job task. She was successful because she used the correct facts to solve her problem at work.

ᴇxᴇʀᴄɪsᴇ
12–5

Directions: Read the following descriptions of work situations. Decide how you would use mathematics to fulfill the job task. Explain your reasoning.

1. Dr. Savari asked you to fill the aquarium in his dental office with water. The aquarium is 20.4 centimeters wide and 30 centimeters long. How much water will fill the aquarium to a depth of 16 centimeters?

   _____

   _____

   _____

2. You are asked to purchase 500 stamps for the office. Forty percent of the stamps are for letters and the rest are for postcards. How many stamps are you purchasing at the rate for postcards?

   _____

   _____

   _____

3. You are required to purchase food for the hospital cafeteria. Mayonnaise in the 12-ounce jar costs $0.56 per ounce. Mayonnaise in the 16-ounce jar costs $9.53. Which is the better value? Explain why.

_____

_____

_____

4. You have estimated that you need 3 hours to finish typing a report. You type 290 words per minute. How many words are in the report?

_____

_____

_____

5. You are asked to estimate the cost of an office party. Food will be $300, entertainment will be $270, drinks are 50% of the cost of the food, and service is 30% of the cost of the food and drinks. The total cost must not go over $1000. Do you think that you are within the budget?

_____

_____

_____

CRITICAL READING

Previewing

Preview this selection. Think about what you already know about this topic. In the space provided, write what you still wish to know.

_____

_____

_____

_____

_____

_____

_____

_____

_____

Questioning

Based on your preview, formulate questions that will help you learn what you still wish to know about the topic.

_____

_____

_____

Reading

Read the following selection from _Saunders Fundamentals for Nursing Assistants_ (pp. 156 to 159).

▼ **Caring Comment**

The very young and the elderly cool off much faster than persons in other age groups. Be certain to provide comfort and warmth for patients who are not comfortable in their environment.

Measuring Body Temperature

Scales

FAHRENHEIT SCALE
a temperature scale with the freezing point at 32° and the boiling point of water at 212°; abbreviated F

There are two scales of measurement you need to know. They are the **Fahrenheit (F)** and the **Celsius** or centigrade (C) scales (Table 12-1). Your health care facility will use one of these scales. A special formula is available if you are asked to convert your reading from one scale to another (see box).

CELSIUS SCALE
a temperature scale with the freezing point at 0° and the boiling point of water at 100°; abbreviated C

Sites for Taking Body Temperature

Body temperature is measured at four sites

The Mouth (Orally). The mouth is the most frequently used site because it is convenient and is comfortable for and accepted by the patient.

TABLE 12–1   Fahrenheit and Celsius Scale Equivalents

Fahrenheit		Celsius
95.9°		35.5°
96.8°		36.0°
97.7°		36.5°
98.6°	Normal	**37.0°**
99.0°		37.2°
99.5°		37.5°
100.4°		38.0°
101.3°		38.5°
102.2°		39.0°
103.1°		39.5°
104.0°		40.0°
104.9°		40.5°

FORMULA TO CONVERT TEMPERATURE MEASUREMENTS FROM ONE SCALE TO THE OTHER

To convert a Fahrenheit reading to a Celsius or centigrade reading, subtract 32 from the Fahrenheit reading and multiply by 5/9.

Example: 97.6° F = ?° C

97.6 − 32.0 = 65.6

$$65.6 \times \frac{5}{9} = \frac{3280}{9} = 36.6° \text{ C}$$

To convert a Celsius or centigrade reading to a Fahrenheit reading, multiply the Celsius reading by 9/5 and add 32.

Example 39.0° C = ?° F

$$39.0 \times \frac{9}{5} = \frac{351.0}{5} = 70.2 + 32.0 = 102.2° \text{ F}$$

The Rectum (Rectally). The rectal temperature is the most accurate representation of the body's temperature. You should measure a rectal temperature in children under the age of 6 or according to the policy of your health care institution. A rectal temperature is measured whenever the patient situation demands it.

RECTUM
the last part of the large intestine that ends at the anal canal

Under the Axilla (Axillary). An axillary temperature is measured in the axilla. This method provides the least accurate measurement.

AXILLA
the armpit

The Ear (Tympanic). A tympanic temperature is measured by a special device that senses the body's temperature at the tympanic membrane (eardrum).

TYMPANIC
pertaining to the eardrum

Whenever the patient has difficulty breathing through the nose, always ask the nurse or supervisor if a rectal body temperature measurement should be taken.

Do not take an oral temperature in the following situations:

- Nasal packing is present.
- The patient is under the age of 6.
- The patient is unconscious.
- Oxygen is being administered
- The patient has a nasogastric tube.
- The patient is confused or disoriented.
- The patient breathes through the mouth
- The patient is paralyzed as a result of a stroke.
- The patient has had surgery or injury of the face, mouth, nose, or neck.

Average Body Temperature by Site

When measured by mouth, the average body temperature is 98.6° F or 37.0° C.
When measured rectally, the average temperature is higher:

- 99.6° F (higher by 1° on the Fahrenheit scale)
- 37.5° C (higher by about .50° on the Celsius scale)

When an axillary (under the arm) measurement is done, the average temperature is lower than the average temperature by mouth.

- 97.6° F (lower by 1° on the Fahrenheit scale)
- 36.5° C (lower by about .50° on the Celsius scale)

TABLE 12–2 Ranges of Normal Body Temperatures by Site

Site	Fahrenheit Scale	Celsius or Centigrade Scale
Oral	97.6° - 99.6°	36.5° - 37.5°
Rectal	98.6° - 100.6°	37.0° - 38.1°
Axillary	96.6° - 98.6°	36.0° - 37.0°

The temperatures given above are only averages. Each site—mouth, rectum, and axillary—has a range of several degrees that are considered to be normal. The ranges are presented in Table 12-2.

Applying

In the space provided, answer your questions.

_____

_____

_____

_____

_____

Evaluating

Were you able to answer all your questions? Yes _____ No _____. Did the selection give you enough information about the topic? Explain.

_____

_____

_____

_____

_____

Check the accuracy of your answers by finding the specific information in the selection.

STUDENT JOURNAL

List what you have learned about using mathematics in the workplace.	How would you apply this knowledge to your study or work in the health fields?

UNIT IV

Applying Critical Thinking Skills to Studying

Successfully preparing for and taking tests is the ultimate goal of all health care students. Unit IV, Applying Critical Thinking Skills to Studying, presents engaging alternatives to the usual study procedures. Chapter 13, Becoming an Active Learner, teaches you the strategies that will motivate you to read your textbooks critically and listen to lectures with utmost concentration. Chapter 14, Creating Your Personal Study Guide, shows you how to develop study techniques that suit your individual needs. Chapter 15, Assessing Your Test-Taking Skills, helps you evaluate your strategies for taking tests. Using the ideas from Unit IV helps you plan for and take tests more competently.

Chapter 13

Becoming an Active Learner

▼ **LEARNING OBJECTIVES**

In this chapter you will learn how to
- Use strategies to enable you to become more involved with the information in your textbooks and lectures.

▼ **PREDICTING VOCABULARY**

Directions: Preview this chapter by finding five words that you recognize but whose precise definition you don't know. Use your background knowledge to write a sentence for each word that predicts the definition of that word.

EXERCISE 13–1

Word 1: _____

Sentence: _____

_____

Word 2: _____

Sentence: _____

_____

Word 3: _____

Sentence: _____

_____

Word 4: _____

Sentence: _____

_____

Word 5: _____

Sentence: _____

_____

When you finish reading this chapter, evaluate the accuracy of your sentences. Make any necessary revisions.

Revisions

_____

_____

_____

_____

_____

_____

_____

_____

_____

▼ UNDERSTANDING ACTIVE LEARNING

Maybe you have been curious about how top students manage to get the best grades. You may have felt that they are doing something differently than you do. Do top students think about old and new facts in a special way? Do they have a certain style for reading their textbooks? What do top students do when they don't understand what they are reading or hearing in class? How do they improve their comprehension so that they can perform better on exams?

The accomplishments of most successful students come from their being active learners. Being an active learner means that you are totally involved in reading and learning the material from your textbooks and lectures. You are not just reading words endlessly to prepare for exams. You are rolling up your sleeves and pitching right in to extract and understand the important information from your textbook and class discussions. Active learners are the students who get the winning grades.

Active learning incorporates all aspects of critical thinking. To be an active learner, you must understand what you are reading in textbooks and hearing in lectures. To be an active learner, you must be able to analyze and synthesize both new and old information. To be an active learner, you must be able to apply information you have read to real-life situations. Finally, to be an active learner, you must be able to evaluate not only the value of the information you are being asked to learn but also your efforts at learning new information.

Directions: Assess your current style as a learner. Read each of the following statements and indicate whether the statement describes your way of learning or not. Check the appropriate response.

EXERCISE **13–2**

1. Before I read a new chapter, I look at the title and try to recall what I already know about the subject. Yes _____ No _____
2. I have some strategies for previewing a chapter before I read it.
   Yes _____ No _____
3. I have a systematic way of determining what I want to learn.
   Yes _____ No _____
4. I am aware of not understanding ideas from my textbooks or lectures.
   Yes _____ No _____
5. I have a method for improving my comprehension of concepts from my textbook or lectures. Yes _____ No _____

   If you answered yes to most of the above statements, you are probably an active learner already. However, if you answered mostly no, it will be worth your while to learn new strategies for active learning.

   Active learning is a four-stage process. In the first stage you think about what you already know about the topic you are studying. In the second stage you decide what you want to learn and then formulate preview questions. In the third stage you devise a means to alert yourself to when you are not understanding information you are reading or hearing during class. In the fourth stage you decide the best way of improving your comprehension.

Directions: Answer the following questions in the spaces provided.

EXERCISE **13–3**

1. Define what it means to you to be an active learner. Be specific.

   _____

   _____

   _____

   _____

2. Give examples of how you would accomplish each of the four stages of active learning. Then compare your ideas with those given in the next section of this chapter.

   _____

   _____

   _____

   _____

   _____

   _____

▼ INTERPRETING ACTIVE LEARNING

Now let's take a closer look at ways to implement each of the four stages of active learning.

Stage One: Activating Your Background Knowledge

The easiest way to learn new information is to associate it with what you already know about the topic. Having a framework for applying new knowledge helps you put these new ideas in a context. Once facts are put in context, they are easier to understand and remember. To activate your background knowledge, look at the chapter title before you begin to read the chapter. Write down all the ideas that come into your head about the chapter title. Do not censor your writing efforts. There are no right or wrong responses. What you want to do is recall any knowledge you already have on the subject. Look at how one reader responded to a chapter titled "Using a Word Processor in the Medical Office."

I am already familiar with using a word processor for my personal and school needs. I use a word processor to do the following:

- *Type my term papers*
- *Type my personal correspondence*
- *Keep my finances straight*
- *Organize my time and create schedules and calendars*
- *Keep my personal appointments straight*
- *Maintain an address and phone book*
- *Keep records of my school grades*

I assume that once I am working in a medical office, I will be using a word processor for many of the same reasons. The chapter "Using a Word Processor in the Medical Office" must discuss most of these functions.

Once the student read the chapter, she felt she had some familiarity with the subject. She was able to relate the new ideas to her background knowledge. Understanding the chapter was less difficult than it would have been had the reader not activated her background knowledge.

EXERCISE
13-4

Directions: Below are some titles for chapters. In the spaces following each title, write briefly what you already know about the titles.

1. The Structure of the Tooth

_____

_____

_____

2. Restraining the Dog

_____

_____

_____

3. Taking Dictation

_____

_____

_____

4. Discharging the Patient

_____

_____

_____

5. Maintaining the Patient's Chart

_____

_____

_____

6. Making Travel Arrangements

_____

_____

_____

7. The Proper Use of the Telephone

_____

_____

_____

8. Animal Nutrition

_____

_____

_____

9. Understanding Medical Orders

_____

_____

_____

10. Using the Proper Dental Instruments

_____

_____

_____

Stage Two: Determining What You Want to Learn and Formulating Questions

To be an active learner, you must be in control of what you want to learn. To determine what you want to learn from your textbook chapter, you must first familiarize yourself with the basic features of the chapter. This means previewing the chapter by paying special attention to the following:

- Chapter title
- Learning objectives
- Chapter introduction
- Italicized terms
- Chapter headings and subheadings
- Illustrations, charts, and graphs
- End-of-chapter summaries
- End-of-chapter questions

Directions: Choose one chapter from this textbook or another textbook. Preview the chapter, focusing on the important features in the chapter. Then think about the answers to the following questions:

1. What is the chapter title?
2. Are there learning objectives for the chapter?
3. Summarize in one sentence the introductory paragraph.
4. What are three italicized terms?
5. List three chapter headings or subheadings.
6. What is the title for an illustration, chart, or graph?
7. Is there an end-of-chapter summary?
8. Are there end-of-chapter questions?

Once you are familiar with the main features of the chapter, you can decide what you want to learn. To determine what you want to learn, try to go beyond basic understanding. Think critically and create questions that will allow you to interpret, apply, and evaluate information. To interpret the information you have read, you can use the following questions:

How does _____ work?

Why does _____ happen?

Why is _____ important?

What are the different solutions for the problem? _____

What is a new plan for _____?

To help you apply the information you have read, you can ask the following questions:

How would I use _____ to solve the problem?

How does _____ apply to my life?

How can _____ be used to _____?

To help you evaluate the information you have read, you can ask the following questions:

Which is the best? _____

What solution should I use and why? _____

_____

How do I rate _____?

Do I agree or disagree and why? _____

_____

Directions: Refer to the chapter you previewed in Exercise 13–5. Formulate a series of questions that will help you decide what it is you want to learn. Try to think of questions that will help you not only understand new facts but also analyze, apply, and evaluate the new material. Write your questions in the space provided.

EXERCISE **13–6**

_____

_____

_____

_____

_____

_____

Stage 3: Being Aware of Not Understanding

Active learners are constantly monitoring their understanding when they are reading a textbook or listening to a lecture. They do not just overlook the fact that they are not comprehending the material being presented. Instead active learners are constantly asking themselves if they are understanding. When reading, active learners may have to ask themselves if they are understanding once or twice a page, depending on how difficult the reading is. Active learners in a classroom ask themselves every few minutes if they are understanding the concepts presented in the lecture. Once these types of self inquiries become a habit, active learners monitor their comprehension almost unconsciously. Alarms go off in their heads when they are not comprehending.

Directions: Think about the best way for you to monitor your comprehension when you read and when you attend lectures. In the space provided, describe how you will alert yourself to not understanding.

_____

_____

_____

_____

_____

Stage 4: Correcting Your Misunderstanding

This last stage in becoming an active learner requires that you use strategies to increase your comprehension once you have determined you are not understanding. Following are some suggestions for correcting your misunderstandings.

- Reread your textbook passage or lecture notes. Sometimes with a second reading, all will come clear. Reading aloud may be helpful, too.
- Look up in a glossary of dictionary any vocabulary words that you do not know. Not knowing important terms is a major reason for not understanding.
- Get further background knowledge on the topic by consulting an encyclopedia or easier text. Insufficient knowledge about the topic can hinder your comprehension.
- Try to rewrite the information in your own words. Writing a summary is a good way to test and improve your understanding of long sentences and complex ideas.

Directions: Below is a list of comprehension problems. Read each problem and decide the best way to solve it. Indicate the best strategy in the space provided. Refer to the above list of suggestions, if necessary.

1. I do not know what half the words on the page mean.

_____

2. My mind wandered when I read that passage.

_____

3. I do not understand what the nonspecific defense mechanisms are.

   _____

4. I am having a hard time visualizing how the blood flows through the heart.

   _____

5. This whole chapter is about protozoa. What does that mean?

   _____

6. This entire chapter was much too technical for me.

   _____

7. By the time I get to the bottom of this very long page, I have forgotten what I read.

   _____

8. Sterilization is a complex process, and I cannot remember all the steps after I have read about them.

   _____

9. What do all these terms relating to the cranial nerves mean?

   _____

10. I cannot figure out the passage on how to use the spirometric equipment.

    _____

▼ APPLYING BECOMING AN ACTIVE LEARNER

When you apply active learning strategies, your comprehension improves because you are thinking about the reading selection. Active learning strategies will help you stay focused while you are reading and retain the information you have read.

Students often complain that they lose concentration while reading textbooks and that when they are finished, they don't understand or remember the information. Applying the four stages of active learning will help students comprehend and retain information.

Directions: Apply the four stages of active learning to the following reading selection from *Computer Concepts and Applications for the Medical Office* (Bonewit-West, pp. 21 to 23).

EXERCISE
13–9

COMPUTER MONITOR

A computer monitor is a bulky and fragile visual display device similar to a television screen. The type of monitor most often used in a microcomputer system is a cathode-ray tube (or CRT). A cathode-ray tube works by spraying electrons onto a viewing screen, under the direction of a magnetic field, to form characters on the screen.

The monitor permits the user to view both a) input and, or more specifically, the data entered into the computer, and b) output, the information produced by the computer as a result of processing. Viewing the input display on the monitor allows the user to check the data for accuracy as it is entered. As an output device the monitor is often used to review information that needs to be viewed briefly and for which a printed copy (hardcopy) is not needed. For example, if a forgetful patient calls your office to inquire when his next appointment is scheduled, you can quickly call up this information, view it on the display screen, and relay it to the patient. The term used to describe the visual display of information on the screen of the monitor is *softcopy*. In summary, softcopy is useful when information is needed immediately and a permanent printed record is not required.

The typical computer monitor used in a medical office has a screen size from 10 to 14 inches across measured diagonally with the range of available screen sizes falling between 5 to 20 inches. Most screens are capable of displaying 80 characters of data horizontally and 25 lines vertically (Fig. 13-1) which provides ample space for working on data and displaying information on the screen.

Resolution

An important area of consideration when working with a computer system is the resolution of the monitor. The term *resolution* refers to the sharpness of the image displayed on the screen. A computer monitor with high resolution produces crisp, clear, easy-to-read characters, while images on a low resolution monitor appear somewhat blurry. As a result, individuals working for a prolonged period of time on a low resolution monitor frequently experience eyestrain and headaches. Resolution is measured in units called picture elements or *pixels*. Pixels are "dot" locations on the screen that can be lit up as needed to display characters and other images. Low resolution monitors are lower in cost and display approximately 320 pixels horizontally and 200 pixels vertically on the screen (320 x 200). High resolution monitors are more expensive but typically display 720 x 350 pixels or more, and are usually preferred for use in the medical office.

Types of Monitors

The CRT may be either a monochrome monitor or a color monitor. A *monochrome monitor* is a display device that exhibits a single-color. Depending upon the brand of monitor, text

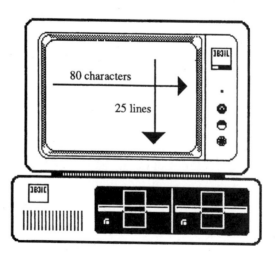

Figure 13–1

Most screens are capable of displaying 80 characters of data horizontally and 25 lines vertically.

is displayed in either white, green, or amber characters on a black background. The best color to use for displaying characters is a matter of individual preference; some individuals prefer working with white characters. While others may prefer green or amber. Monochrome monitors are preferred for those tasks involving the entry of text because they provide better resolution for letters and numbers than do color monitors. In addition, color monitors are much heavier and more expensive than monochrome monitors of the same size. *Color monitors*, on the other hand, display text and graphics in a variety of colors, which is particularly useful when working with charts, graphs, and pictures. It is important to understand, however, that the colors displayed on the screen can be only printed in color if the computer system includes a color printer.

Monitor Controls

Located on either the front or side of the monitor are three important controls which are used to operate and adjust the display screen. The first of these is the *on/off switch*, either a pull-knob or a push-button. When the monitor is turned on, an indicator light comes on denoting that the monitor is receiving power and is ready for use.

There are two controls for adjusting the viewing screen: the brightness control and the contrast control. These controls work much like the same controls on a television set. The *brightness control* allows you to increase or decrease the intensity of the images on the screen. This control should be adjusted until the background just disappears, which provides a good balance between screen and character brightness. If a monitor is left on for long periods of time while not being used, images on the screen will start to "burn in" and the screen may be permanently damaged. To prevent this from happening, the brightness control should be turned down when you are not using the computer, but leaving it on for long periods.

The *contrast control* is used to adjust the screen for comfortable viewing. Contrast refers to the degree of difference between the light and dark areas on the display screen. For example, if you are working with a monochrome monitor that displays white characters on a black background, the contrast would be the amount of difference that exists between the characters (light area) and the background (dark area). Too much contrast makes it uncomfortable to look at the characters on the screen, while not enough contrast results in difficulty in viewing the characters. Because of individual viewing preferences, you should adjust both the brightness and contrast control when first beginning work on the computer to find the setting that works best for your viewing comfort.

Care and Maintenance

The monitor should rest on a flat, stable surface, such as a table or on top of the main computer unit itself. The monitor should be placed so the top of the screen is at eye level or just below eye level to prevent back and neck tension. To avoid glare, the monitor should be positioned so that the screen does not reflect bright light which could result in eye strain. For example, positioning the monitor directly in front of a bright window causes a distracting reflection on the screen. Subdued overhead lighting is considered best for computer use because it causes the least amount of glare. Glare filters are available to help reduce unavoidable reflections such as from bright overhead fluorescent lights. A glare filter is a transparent covering that fits over the front of the screen similar to placing a camera filter over the lens of a camera.

There are a number of ventilation slots on the top of computer monitors which allow heat to escape. To prevent overheating, never place anything (not even a piece of paper) on top of the monitor.

Monitors collect dust and dirt over a period of time and therefore, must be properly maintained. The screen should be cleaned with a household glass cleaner applied with a clean, lint-free cloth or paper towel. The glass cleaner should *not* be sprayed directly on the screen as it may run down into the inside of the case and damage the electrical circuits. The outside casing of the monitor should periodically be wiped with a damp, lint-free cloth to remove dust and dirt. Aerosol sprays, solvents, and abrasives should not be used to clean the casing as they can damage the finish.

Answer the following questions:

Stage 1 What do you already know about your topic?

_____

_____

_____

_____

Stage 2 What do you want to learn about the topic? Formulate preview questions.

_____

_____

_____

_____

Stage 3 Check your comprehension. What information are you not understanding?

_____

_____

_____

_____

Stage 4 How can you improve your understanding of the selection?

_____

_____

_____

_____

▼ EVALUATING BECOMING AN ACTIVE LEARNER

When you have finished reading an assignment or listening to a lecture, you should assess your understanding of the information. Evaluating what you still need to learn is an essential component of active learning. You first have to identify the concepts and facts you have difficulty comprehending. Then you can decide what learning strategies need to be improved so that you can better understand the assigned reading or lecture material.

Directions: Look at your answers in Exercise 13–9. Evaluate your ability to apply the four stages of active learning. Next to each stage, write your assessment of how you can improve your ability to understand and retain information.

EXERCISE 13–10

Stage 1

_____

_____

_____

Stage 2

_____

_____

_____

Stage 3

_____

_____

_____

Stage 4

_____

_____

_____

CRITICAL READING

Previewing

Preview this selection. Think about what you already know about this topic. In the space provided, write what you still wish to know.

_____

_____

_____

_____

Questioning

Based on your preview, formulate questions that will help you learn what you still wish to know about the topic.

_____

_____

_____

_____

Reading

Read the following selection from *Saunders Fundamentals for Nursing Assistants* (Polaski and Warner, pp. 77-80).

Caring Comments

Your gestures and expressions give the listener as much information as your words. The patient and others receive an accurate picture of your feelings when your body language matches what you say.

You will be more successful using your new communication skills when you have a positive, willing attitude.

THE ESSENTIAL PARTS OF COMMUNICATION

COMMUNICATION
an exchange of information

INTERACTION
communication between two or more people

KNOWLEDGE BASE
the basis of one's information and understanding

Communication is an exchange of information. When information is exchanged between people, an **interaction** occurs. Each interaction is based on three important points:

- **Knowledge base**—The knowledge we acquire while growing and maturing is called a **knowledge base.** We use our knowledge base to create questions, find answers, and make decisions. We bring our personal knowledge base to every interaction we have with another person.
- **Feelings**—The feelings of the people involved in any interaction color the messages and responses they use. Feelings give personal identity to any interaction. Most times, we are not aware of how much our feelings contribute to an interaction.
- **Past experiences**—Past experience helps us learn to handle events realistically. Any experience, whether positive or negative, helps shape our future interactions with others.

In order for communication to occur, the following four essential parts are necessary:

Sender
Message
Receiver
Feedback

These four parts occur in a series of events called the **communication process** (Fig. 13–2). The exchange of information occurs when all parts of the communication process are completed. The process is repeated many times in the course of an interaction. The act of communicating involves at least two people, a sender and a receiver.

The Sender

The sender is the person who begins or continues an interaction by "sending" information to another person. The sender uses the spoken or written word and body language (e.g., nodding the head or making a fist) to give the information.

As an example, imagine two housemates, Sarah and Kate. Sarah comes into the kitchen in the morning and begins to speak. Sarah is the sender.

The Message

The information that the sender expresses is the message. It may be a question or a statement. The message is sent through sound (for example, words or music) or body language.

Sarah's message is "I'll be home late tonight."

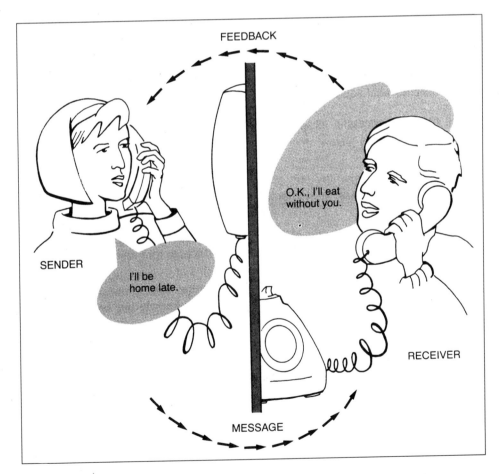

Figure 13–2
The communication process.

The Receiver

The receiver is the person who "gets" (hears and sees) the message from the sender. A receiver pays attention and is a good listener.

The receiver of Sarah's message is her housemate, Kate.

FEEDBACK

when the receiver in the communication process repeats the information the sender sent (or otherwise acknowledges it) to make sure the message is clear and well understood

Feedback

The receiver listens to the message and understands it. The receiver then repeats the sender's message or otherwise acknowledges it to make sure it was understood correctly.

In the kitchen, Kate gives Sarah **feedback** by saying, "O.K., if you're going to be late, I won't bother waiting, I'll go on and eat without you."

VERBAL COMMUNICATION

VERBAL COMMUNICATION

the use of words or other sounds such as music or groans to exchange information

Verbal communication, the most common way people communicate, involves the use of words or sounds. To take part in verbal communication, a person must possess the ability to send and receive messages. Speaking and writing are two ways most people learn to send messages. The spoken word is effective only when the receiver of the message can hear and the sender can speak. A speech therapist is someone who is trained to help people who have difficulty speaking. The written word is effective only for receivers who can see or have someone read the message to them. Most of your communications with patients are verbal. Express all messages to patients as clearly as possible and listen carefully to their feedback. Always introduce yourself when you first care for a patient. Because so many different care givers contact the patient during a shift, you may need to reintroduce yourself several times.

Communication Helpers

Communication helpers are ways to make the communication process better so that the message is more likely to be understood. Pay attention to what the patient says. You should look at patients when they speak to you. Not all words have the same meaning to every person, so observation of the patient's body language is necessary.

Listening

LISTENING

paying attention; hearing a message with thoughtful attention

Paying attention tells patients you are interested in their message. Most patients send a clear message that you, as the receiver, will understand. Remember that some people find it difficult to express their feelings and needs in words. **Listening** is an important part of communication.

A General Lead

A general lead helps patients expand on a statement they have made. By simply saying "Oh?" or "Go on" or "Hmm," you are telling patients that you are an attentive listener and wish to continue the communication. For example, a patient, during a bath, might say to you, "My daughter called this morning and told me she's having problems in school." You could say, "Go on." The patient might reply, "She knows she has to go to school, but she misses me and I feel she is not doing well because I'm sick." By using a general lead, you might learn information that will help the nurse in planning the patient's care.

A Broad Opening Statement

When you wish to encourage patients to introduce a particular topic of concern or interest to them, use a broad opening statement. This allows patients to choose the direction of the interaction. You are allowing patients to select the topics they wish to discuss. For example, you might notice that a patient is especially quiet today. You could say, "You seem quiet today. Is there something you would like to talk about?" Another example would be to pick up on something the patient mentioned earlier in the shift. Perhaps the patient told you several times of feeling angry. You could say, "You seem to be angry about what is happening to you. Let's take this time to talk about your feelings."

Reflection

When you feel the need to explore information with your patients, try a technique called reflection. Use key words your patients say to reflect a main idea back to them. Reflection allows patients to expand on their original statement and helps communication about a topic important to them. When a person says, "I'm feeling really sad today," you can respond. "You're feeling sad?" Avoid using *only* reflection, however, because, if it is used too often, patients may ask if you are listening to them.

Silence

Silence is a useful helper. A few moments of silence can help patients gather their thoughts so they can state what they need. Be careful not to remain silent for extended periods of time though. When you remain silent for short periods of time, patients are supported by your presence and become more trusting. It becomes easier for them to exchange information when they sense you truly care. You may feel comfortable with silence in your own home but find it difficult to use effectively with patients. Keep trying. When you have become comfortable with using silence, your role as a helping care giver is enhanced.

Clarification

Ask patients to clarify (make more clear) any message you do not understand. Always make sure the message is what the patients intend. When you are not sure of the message, you are responsible for asking patients to help you understand. If a person tells you, "I have pain when I bend my arm," you can clarify by using a statement like, "Bend your arm and point to where the pain is."

Applying

In the space provided, answer your questions.

_____

_____

_____

_____

_____

_____

_____

Evaluating

Were you able to answer all your questions? Yes _____ No _____. Did the selection give you enough information about the topic? Explain.

_____

_____

_____

_____

_____

_____

_____

Check the accuracy of your answers by finding the specific information in the selection.

STUDENT JOURNAL

List what you have learned about becoming an active learner	How would you apply this knowledge to your study or work in the health fields?

Chapter 14

Creating a Personal Study Guide

▼ LEARNING OBJECTIVES

In this chapter you will learn how to
- Design a personal study guide to enable you to become an active learner

▼ PREDICTING VOCABULARY

Directions: Preview this chapter by finding five words that you recognize but whose precise definition you don't know. Use your background knowledge to write a sentence for each word that predicts the definition of that word.

Word 1: _____

Sentence: _____

_____

Word 2: _____

Sentence: _____

_____

Word 3: _____

Sentence: _____

_____

Word 4: _____

Sentence: _____

_____

Word 5: _____

Sentence: _____

_____

When you finish reading this chapter, evaluate the accuracy of your sentences. Make any necessary revisions.

Revisions

_____

_____

_____

_____

_____

_____

_____

_____

_____

▼ UNDERSTANDING THE PERSONAL STUDY GUIDE

Sol prides himself on being a diligent health care student. He believes that he reads his textbooks well, and he takes careful notes even though he finds the note-taking process tiresome. When a test is announced, he begins to organize his time schedule so that he has plenty of time to study. Much of his study time is spent rereading the appropriate textbook chapters and going over his lecture notes. While Sol understands the necessity for all his effort, many times he has wished there was a more interesting and efficient way to prepare for exams. While his grades have been good enough, he feels that reading, rereading, and rereading again is a boring and passive way of learning new material. Sol wants a more individual and active way of studying for tests.

After much thought, Sol decides that he will design his own personal study guide. The guide will enable him to organize the information he needs to learn in a way that will make studying easier and more enjoyable. He also thinks that writing a personal study guide will be a great way to help him understand, interpret, apply, and evaluate the new ideas he needs to learn. Following are some of the features that Sol feels the personal study guide must have.

1. Easy to carry
2. Lend itself to efficient organization
3. For his personal reading only
4. A section for his prereading and previewing activities
5. A section for his postreading activities
6. A section for important points that will appear on the test
7. A section for questions he needs to research further
8. A section for his impressions and observations
9. A section for vocabulary he needs to learn

EXERCISE 14–2

Directions: In the space below, list all the features you would need for your own personal study guide.

_____

_____

_____

_____

_____

_____

_____

_____

_____

_____

_____

▼ INTERPRETING THE PERSONAL STUDY GUIDE

Sol decides that for his personal study guide a looseleaf binder divided into five sections will be best. He will use one binder for each of his school subjects. He will use the first section for his previewing section. This section will include notes he makes linking his background knowledge of the subject to the new knowledge, questions he makes from chapter boldface headings, and his critical thinking questions on what information he would like to learn. He will use the second section for his notes after he reads the chapter. These notes will include his correction of any misunderstandings he had about information in the chapter during the prereading phase. The third section will contain any questions he has about the material in the chapter. This third section will also include any vocabulary words he still needs to learn. The fourth section will include any of Sol's personal observations and impressions about the material he has read and needs to learn. The fifth section will contain all the important points he believes will appear on the test.

Sol heads the five sections as follows:

Section 1: Prereading Ideas
Section 2: Postreading Ideas
Section 3: Questions and New Vocabulary
Section 4: Personal Observations and Thoughts
Section 5: Important Facts for the Test

The following is an example of Sol's prereading and postreading entries. This example also shows the writing format Sol has decided to use for the other three sections. Note that Sol is writing for himself so he does not feel it is necessary to write complete sentences. However, he realizes that he will have to be able to understand what his writing means days or weeks later.

PREREADING IDEAS

I know body tries for fluid balance. That's why I get thirsty. Some chemistry appears to be involved (sodium and potassium). What are electrolytes? My guess is that the hypothalamus will play a big role in fluid regulation. What is the mechanism? I need to learn more about ADH. What are the two main fluid compartments? What is fluid balance? How is electrolyte balance affected by fluid balance?

POSTREADING IDEAS

Two thirds of body fluid found within cells. One third found in tissue space between cells, blood plasma, lymph, cerebrospinal fluid. Normally the amount of fluid we ingest is equal to the amount we lose from the kidneys, skin, lungs, and digestive tract. Hypothalamus regulates thirst center. ADH regulates the volume of urine and is produced by hypothalamus. Electrolytes—found in fluids and form ions. Electrolytes become more concentrated or diluted depending on the amount of body fluid. Calcium, phosphate, chloride, and magnesium—other electrolytes.

Directions: Following is a list of ideas and facts taken from Sol's textbook chapter (see Exercise 14–5). Decide in what section of his personal study guide Sol should put the idea or fact. Indicate the appropriate section in the space provided.

EXERCISE
14–3

1. What are chloride ions? Section _____

2. I remember that athletes have a problem with electrolytes when they are playing a vigorous game. Section _____

3. Professor Clark says we need to know about the hormones that affect the kidneys. Section _____

4. The chapter says that when the sodium concentration is too high, we feel thirsty. That explains why I drink gallons after eating a bag of chips. Section _____

5. When I first looked at the chapter, I did not realize the numerous functions magnesium has. Section _____

6. I think much of this chapter will deal with fluid intake and output. Section _____

7. What are the intercellular and extracellular compartments? I cannot visualize them. Section _____

8. Professor Clark claims homeostasis is important. I must learn the chart for the test. Section _____

9. When I first looked at the chapter, I did not see that the hypothalamus regulates both fluid intake and output. Section _____

10. I somehow never realized that water is contained in the solid foods we eat and must be considered when we determine our daily intake of fluid. Section _____

EXERCISE 14-4

Directions: In the space provided, describe the ideal way of organizing your personal study guide. Specify the number of sections and section headings. Feel free to use some of Sol's ideas if you think they will satisfy your needs.

_____

_____

_____

_____

_____

_____

_____

_____

_____

_____

_____

▼ **APPLYING THE PERSONAL STUDY GUIDE**

The first time Sol makes and uses his personal study guide is to prepare for his test on fluid regulation. Even though he has not taken the test yet, he thinks that making the personal study guide has been more rewarding and enjoyable than his old method of study. He feels more in control of the material and considers himself more actively involved with his studying than previously. Now it is your turn to try out the personal study guide.

Directions: Following is an excerpt from *Introduction to Human Anatomy and Physiology* (Solomon, pp. 241-244). Using your format or Sol's format, create a personal study guide in the space provided, after you have previewed and read the selection. Use headings and write in a few ideas under each heading.

EXERCISE **14-5**

REGULATION OF FLUIDS AND ELECTROLYTES

Chapter Outline
   I. The body has two main fluid compartments
   II. Fluid intake must equal fluid output
      A. The hypothalamus regulates fluid intake
      B. The hypothalamus also regulates fluid output
   III. Electrolyte balance is affected by fluid balance
      A. Sodium is the major extracellular cation
      B. Potassium is the major intracellular cation
      C. Other major electrolytes include calcium, phosphate, chloride, and magnesium

Learning Objectives
After you have studied this chapter, you should be able to:
1. Identify the fluid compartments of the body.
2. Summarize the principal routes for fluid input and fluid output.
3. Describe how fluid input and output are regulated.
4. Define electrolyte balance and identify the functions of six major electrolytes.
5. Describe the mechanisms responsible for sodium and potassium homeostasis.

Fluid balance is critical to homeostasis. Whether you drink a pint of water or a gallon, whether you are on a salt-restricted diet or eat a bag of potato chips, the fluid and salt content of your body must be kept within strict limits. To keep the quantities of these substances steady, the body must replace water and salt losses and excrete excesses. Normal body function, and even survival, depend upon homeostasis of body fluids.

The term **body fluid** refers to the water in the body and the substances dissolved in it. Among the most important components of body fluid are **electrolytes** (ee-**lek'**-trow-lites), compounds such as salts that form ions (electrically charged particles) in solution. Most organic compounds dissolved in the body fluid are nonelectrolytes, compounds that do not form ions. Examples of nonelectrolytes in the body fluid are glucose and urea.

The Body Has Two Main Fluid Compartments

The human body is about 60% water by weight. Water and electrolytes are distributed in certain regions, or compartments. The two principal compartments are the **intracellular compartment** and the **extracellular compartment.** About two thirds of the body fluid is found in the intracellular compartment, that is, within cells (Fig. 14-1). This fluid is referred to as intracellular fluid. The remaining third is located outside the cells in the extracellular compartment. This extracellular fluid includes the tissue fluid, also called interstitial fluid, found in the tissue spaces between cells; the blood plasma and lymph; the cerebrospinal fluid; and all other fluids in the body.

Fluid constantly moves from one compartment to another. However, in a healthy person, the volume of fluid in each compartment remains about the same. The movement of fluid from one compartment to another depends upon blood pressure and osmotic concentration. Recall that blood pressure forces fluid out of the blood at the arterial ends of capillaries. When it leaves the blood, this fluid is called tissue fluid. Excess tissue fluid re-

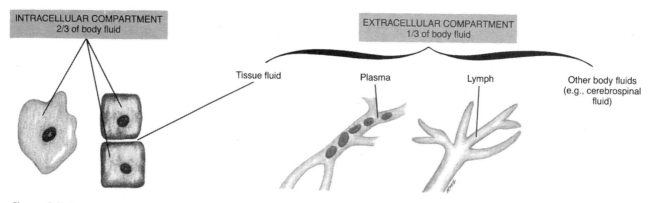

Figure 14-1
Fluid compartments

turns to the blood at the venous ends of capillaries because of osmotic pressure. (Plasma proteins in the plasma exert a pulling force on fluid.) Excess tissue fluid is also returned to the blood by way of the lymphatic system. Fluid movement between the intracellular and extracellular compartments occurs mainly as a result of changes in osmotic pressure.

Important differences in composition exist between the intracellular fluid and the extracellular fluid. For example, sodium ion concentration is much higher in the extracellular fluid than in the intracellular fluid. In contrast, potassium ion concentration is much higher in the extracellular fluid. To maintain these differences in ion distribution, cells must pump specific kinds of ions into or out of the cell. This is a form of cellular work known as active transport.

Fluid Intake Must Equal Fluid Output

Normally, fluid input equals fluid output, so the total amount of fluid in the body remains constant (Fig. 14-2). We ingest about 2500 milliliters (ml) of water each day in the foods we eat and liquids we drink. This water is absorbed from the digestive tract into the blood. Water is also produced during catabolic processes. Most fluid (about 1500 ml per day) is discharged by the kidneys. Fluid is also lost through the skin, lungs, and the digestive tract.

When fluid output is greater than fluid input, dehydration occurs. Dehydration can result from not drinking enough fluid, from profuse sweating, or as a result of vomiting or diarrhea.

The Hypothalamus Regulates Fluid Intake

Fluid intake is regulated by the hypothalamus. Dehydration raises the osmotic pressure of the blood (when there is less fluid, the blood is saltier). The increased osmotic pressure stimulates the **thirst center** in the hypothalamus (Fig. 14-3). This results in the sensation of thirst and the desire to drink fluids. Dehydration also leads to a decrease in saliva secretion that results in dryness in the mouth and throat. This dryness also signals thirst. We feel thirsty when total body fluid is decreased more than 1 to 2%.

The Hypothalamus also Regulates Fluid Output

The kidneys are primarily responsible for fluid output. This output is regulated by ADH (antidiuretic hormone). Recall that ADH, produced by the hypothalamus and secreted by the posterior lobe of the pituitary gland, regulates the volume of urine.

When the body begins to dehydrate, ADH secretion increases. This occurs because the plasma becomes saltier when the volume of water in the body decreases. Special receptors in the hypothalamus signal the posterior pituitary to release more ADH. The ADH makes

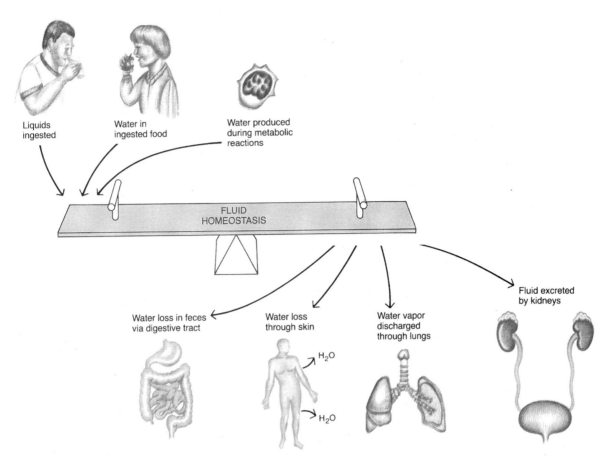

Figure 14–2
Fluid intake and output.

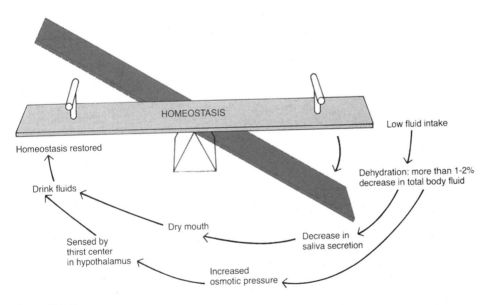

Figure 14–3
Regulation of fluid intake.

the distal tubules and collecting ducts in the kidneys more permeable to water. More water is reabsorbed into the blood, and only a small volume of concentrated urine is excreted.

When blood volume increases, less ADH is secreted. Less water is reabsorbed, and a large volume of dilute urine is excreted. In this way, fluid homeostasis is restored.

Electrolyte Balance Is Affected by Fluid Balance

Normally, a person obtains adequate amounts of electrolytes in the food and fluid ingested. When the amounts of the various electrolytes taken into the body equal the amounts lost, the body is in **electrolyte balance.** Because electrolytes are dissolved in the body fluid, electrolyte balance and fluid balance are interdependent. When the fluid content decreases, the electrolytes become more concentrated; when fluid content increases, electrolytes are more diluted.

Electrolytes produce positively and negatively charged ions. Positively charged ions are referred to as cations; negatively charged ions are anions. Among the important cations in the body fluid are sodium, potassium, calcium, hydrogen, magnesium, and iron. Important anions include chloride and phosphate.

Sodium Is the Major Extracellular Cation

About 90% of the extracellular cations are **sodium** ions. Sodium is needed to transmit impulses in nervous and muscle tissue. Low sodium concentration can cause headache, mental confusion, rapid heart rate, low blood pressure, and even circulatory shock. Severe sodium depletion can result in coma.

Sodium concentration is adjusted mainly by regulating the amount of water in the body. When the sodium concentration is too high, we feel thirsty and drink water. In addition, sodium concentration is regulated by the hormone aldosterone secreted by the adrenal cortex. Aldosterone stimulates the distal convoluted tubules and collecting ducts to increase their reabsorption of sodium.

Potassium Is the Major Intracellular Cation

Most of the cations in the intracellular fluid are **potassium** ions. These cations are important in nervous and muscle tissue function. Potassium ions are also important in maintaining the fluid volume within cells, and they help regulate acid-base levels (pH). An abnormally low level of potassium may cause mental confusion, fatigue, and cramps, and it may affect the heart. When the potassium concentration is too high, nerve impulses are not effectively transmitted and the strength of muscle contraction decreases. In fact, a high potassium concentration can weaken the heart and lead to death from heart failure.

When the concentration of potassium ions is too high, potassium ions are secreted from the blood into the renal tubules, and the ions are excreted in the urine. This is due to a direct effect of the potassium ions on the tubules. A high potassium ion concentration also stimulates aldosterone secretion. The aldosterone further stimulates secretion of potassium. Loss of large numbers of potassium ions in the urine brings the potassium concentration in the body back to normal. When the potassium concentration becomes too low, aldosterone secretion decreases, and potassium secretion decreases almost to zero.

Other Major Electrolytes Include Calcium, Phosphate, Chloride, and Magnesium

Calcium is found mainly in the extracellular fluid. **Phosphate** is the most abundant intracellular anion. Calcium and phosphate are both important components of bone and teeth. Calcium is also important in blood clotting, transmission of neural impulses, and muscle contraction. Phosphate is needed to make ATP, DNA, and RNA. The concentrations of calcium and phosphate are regulated by parathyroid hormone and calcitonin.

Chloride ions are the most abundant extracellular anions. These ions can diffuse easily across plasma membranes. Their movement is closely linked to the movement of sodium ions. Chloride helps regulate differences in osmotic pressure between fluid compartments and is also important in pH balance. The hormone aldosterone indirectly regulates chloride concentration.

Magnesium ions are cations found mainly in the intracellular fluid and in bone. They are important in production of bone and teeth and play a role in neural transmission and muscle contraction. The hormone aldosterone increases reabsorption of magnesium ions by the kidneys.

Create your personal study guide here:

_____

_____

_____

_____

_____

_____

_____

_____

_____

_____

_____

_____

_____

_____

_____

_____

_____

_____

_____

_____

_____

▼ EVALUATING THE PERSONAL STUDY GUIDE

Your personal study guide will be only as good as your test results. Sol is pleased with his personal study guide, since he has scored a letter grade higher than he usually does. He feels that the extra effort was well worth the results. However, to determine whether you are on the right track with your personal study guide, you must compare the information in your personal study guide with the questions that were asked on the test. You must also see if your answers on the test corresponded to what you wrote in your personal study guide.

Directions: Below is a checklist you can use to evaluate the effectiveness of your personal study guide. After you have used your personal study guide in a real testing situation, answer the following questions by indicating yes or no. If the majority of your answers are yes, you have designed an adequate personal study guide. If the majority of your answers are no, you may need to restructure the appropriate parts of your personal study guide.

Checklist

1. Did my personal study guide cover the major areas that were on the test? Yes _____ No _____
2. Did I accurately define all the important terms in my personal study guide? Yes _____ No _____
3. Did I correctly clear up all misconceptions I may have had when I previewed the chapter? Yes _____ No _____
4. Did I find out the correct answers to all my questions? Yes _____ No _____
5. Were my personal observations helpful in giving me a deeper understanding of the topic? Yes _____ No _____
6. Did I accurately answer all my heading questions? Yes _____ No _____
7. Did linking my background knowledge to the new information enable me to understand the new facts better? Yes _____ No _____
8. Did my personal study guide make me feel more involved with the topic? Yes _____ No _____
9. Was I able to decipher my writing days or weeks later? Yes _____ No _____
10. Were my test scores better? Yes _____ No _____

CRITICAL READING

Previewing

Preview this selection. Think about what you already know about this topic. In the space provided, write what you still need to know.

_____

_____

_____

_____

Questioning

Based on your preview, formulate questions that will help you learn what you still need to know about the topic. Use the space provided.

_____

_____

_____

_____

_____

Reading

Read the following selection from *Introduction to Human Anatomy and Physiology* (Solomon, pp. 233-236).

Urine Is Produced by Filtration, Reabsorption, and Secretion

Urine formation involves three processes: (1) glomerular filtration; (2) tubular reabsorption; and (3) tubular secretion (Fig. 14–4).

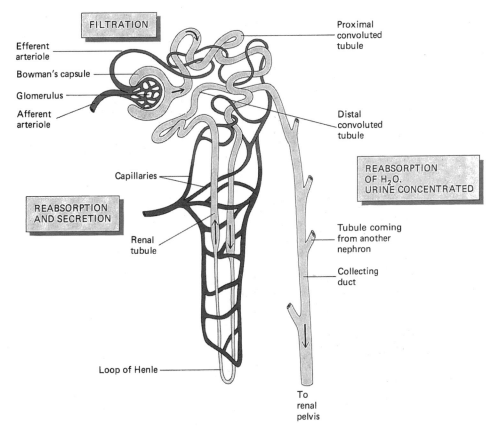

Figure 14–4

Urine is produced by filtration, reabsorption, and secretion.

Glomerular Filtration Is Not a Selective Process

The first step in urine production is **glomerular filtration.** The afferent arteriole is larger in diameter than the efferent arteriole, so blood enters the glomerulus more rapidly than it can leave. This causes the blood pressure to be higher in the glomerular capillaries than in other capillaries. The high pressure forces plasma and substances dissolved in the plasma out of the capillaries and into Bowman's capsule.

The filtrate consists of blood plasma containing small, dissolved molecules. Glomerular filtration is not a selective process. Useful substances such as glucose, amino acids, and salts are present in the filtrate.

Blood cells and proteins are too large to pass through the walls of the capillary and capsule. When blood cells or proteins do appear in the urine, they are signs of a problem with glomerular filtration.

Almost 25% of the cardiac output is delivered to the kidneys each minute, so every 4 minutes the kidneys receive a volume of blood equal to the total volume of blood in the body. Every 24 hours about 180 liters (45 gallons) of filtrate are produced. Common sense suggests that we could not excrete urine at the rate of 45 gallons per day. If we were losing fluid that quickly, dehydration would become a life-threatening problem within a few moments.

Tubular Reabsorption and Secretion Are Selective Processes

Dehydration does not normally occur because about 99% of the filtrate is returned to the blood by **tubular reabsorption.** This leaves only about 1.5 liters to be excreted as urine during a 24-hour period. Tubular reabsorption is the job of the renal tubules and collecting ducts.

Unlike glomerular filtration, tubular reabsorption is highly selective. Wastes, surplus salts, and excess water are kept as part of the filtrate. Glucose, amino acids, and other needed substances are reabsorbed into the blood.

A few substances are actively **secreted** from the blood in the peritubular capillaries into the renal tubules. Tubular secretion is important in regulating the potassium and hydrogen ion concentrations in the blood. Some toxic substances and certain drugs, such as penicillin, are removed from the body by tubular secretion.

Urine Consists Mainly of Water

By the time the filtrate reaches the ureter, its composition has been carefully adjusted. Useful materials have been returned to the blood while wastes and excess materials have been cleared from the blood. The adjusted filtrate is called **urine.** It is composed of about 96% water, 2.5% nitrogen wastes (mainly urea), 1.5% salts, and traces of other substances.

Healthy urine is sterile. However, urine rapidly decomposes when exposed to bacterial action, forming ammonia and other products. The ammonia causes diaper rash in infants.

Urine Volume Is Regulated by ADH

When you drink a large amount of water, your kidneys produce a large volume of urine. Water is absorbed from the digestive tract into the blood. Excess water is removed from the blood by the kidneys. When you drink too little water, only a small volume of urine is produced. By regulating urine volume, the body maintains a steady volume and composition of blood.

The kidney receives information about the state of the blood indirectly (Fig. 14-5). When fluid intake is low, the body begins to dehydrate. When the volume of the blood decreases, the concentration of dissolved salts is greater, causing an increase in the osmotic pressure of the blood. Specialized receptors in the brain, heart, and in certain large blood vessels are sensitive to such change. The posterior lobe of the pituitary gland responds by releasing antidiuretic hormone (ADH). This hormone serves as a

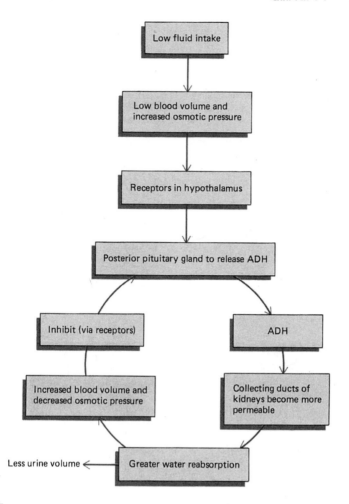

Figure 14–5

Regulation of urine volume reflects the blood volume and osmotic pressure. When the body is dehydrated, the hormone ADH increases the permeability of the collecting ducts to water. More water is reabsorbed, and only a small volume of concentrated urine is produced.

chemical messenger carrying information from the brain to the distal convoluted tubules and collecting ducts of the kidneys. It causes the walls of these ducts to become much more permeable to water, so more water is reabsorbed into the blood. Blood volume increases, and homeostasis of fluid volume is restored. Only a small amount of concentrated urine is produced.

On the other hand, when a great deal of fluid is consumed, the blood becomes diluted and its osmotic pressure falls. Release of ADH by the pituitary gland decreases. This reduces the amount of water reabsorbed from the distal tubules and collecting ducts. As a result, a large volume of dilute urine is produced.

When the pituitary gland does not produce enough ADH, water is not efficiently reabsorbed from the ducts. This results in the production of a large volume of urine. This condition is called diabetes insipidus (not to be confused with the more common disorder, diabetes mellitus). An individual with severe diabetes insipidus may excrete up to 25 quarts of urine each day and must drink almost continually to offset this fluid loss.

ADH regulates the excretion of water by the kidneys. Salt excretion is regulated by hormones, mainly aldosterone, secreted by the adrenal glands.

Coffee, tea, and alcoholic beverages contain chemicals called diuretics that increase urine volume. Diuretics inhibit reabsorption of water. Some diuretics inhibit secretion of ADH; others act directly on the tubules in the kidneys.

The Kidneys Help Maintain Homeostasis

The kidneys are vital in maintaining homeostasis. Their functions include:

1. Excretion of metabolic wastes such as water, urea, and uric acid.
2. Disposal of excess water and salts.
3. Regulation of acid-base (pH) level of blood and body fluids. Acids and bases that are not needed are excreted in the urine.
4. Secretion of regulatory substances. The kidneys secrete the enzyme renin, which is important in regulating blood pressure. They also secrete a hormone (erythropoietin) that regulates production of red blood cells.

Urine Is Transported by Ducts and Stored in the Bladder

Urine passes from the kidneys through the paired ureters, ducts about 25 centimeters (cm) (10 inches) long, which conduct it to the urinary bladder. Urine is forced along through the ureter by peristaltic contractions.

The urinary bladder is a temporary storage sac for urine. The bladder is lined with a mucous membrane that (like the stomach) has folds called rugae. This lining and smooth muscle in its wall permit the bladder to stretch so that it can hold up to 800 milliliters (ml) (about a pint and a half) of urine.

When urine leaves the bladder, it flows through the urethra, a duct leading to the outside of the body. In the male, the urethra is lengthy and passes through the prostate gland and the penis. Semen, as well as urine, is transported through the male urethra. In the female, the urethra is short and transports only urine. Its opening to the outside is just above the opening into the vagina. Bladder infections are more common in females than males because the long male urethra is a barrier to bacterial invasion.

Urination Empties the Bladder

The process of emptying the bladder and expelling urine is referred to as urination, or micturition (mik'-tyoo-**rish**'-un). When the volume of urine in the bladder reaches about 300 ml, special nerve endings in the bladder wall are stimulated. These receptors send neural messages to the spinal cord, initiating a urination reflex. This reflex contracts the bladder wall and also relaxes the internal urethral sphincter, a ring of smooth muscle at the upper end of the urethra. These actions stimulate a conscious desire to urinate.

If the time and place are appropriate, the external urethral sphincter, located a short distance below the internal sphincter, is voluntarily relaxed, allowing urination to occur. Voluntary control of urination cannot be exerted by an immature nervous system. That is why most babies under the age of 2 automatically urinate every time the bladder fills.

Applying

In the space provided, answer your questions.

_____

_____

_____

_____

_____

Evaluation

Were you able to answer all your questions? Yes _____ No _____
Did the selection give you enough information about the topic? Explain.

_____

_____

_____

_____

_____

_____

Check the accuracy of your answers by finding the specific information in the selection.

STUDENT JOURNAL

List what you have learned about creating a personal study guide.	How would you apply this knowledge to your study or work in the health fields?

Chapter 15

Assessing Your Test-Taking Skills

▼ **LEARNING OBJECTIVES**

In this chapter you learn how to
- Assess your test-taking skills
- Improve your strategies for preparing for and taking tests

▼ **PREDICTING VOCABULARY**

Directions: Preview this chapter by finding five words that you recognize but whose precise definition you don't know. Use your background knowledge to write a sentence for each word that predicts the definition of that word.

E X E R C I S E 15–1

Word 1: _____

Sentence: _____

_____

Word 2: _____

Sentence: _____

_____

Word 3: _____

Sentence: _____

_____

Word 4: _____

Sentence: _____

_____

Word 5: _____

Sentence: _____

_____

When you finish reading this chapter, evaluate the accuracy of your sentences. Make any necessary revisions.

Revisions

_____

_____

_____

_____

_____

_____

_____

_____

_____

_____

▼ UNDERSTANDING ASSESSING YOUR TEST-TAKING SKILLS

Matthew studied for several hours for his chemistry exam. He thought he should do well on the test because he had spent time preparing for it. However, when he saw the exam questions, he panicked and realized that he had studied the wrong information. How did this happen?

Lisa went into the exam feeling confident. She knew the material. She started with question 1 and wrote for 30 minutes. The test session was 60 minutes and she had to complete three more questions in the remaining 30 minutes. Lisa never reached question 4; therefore the highest her score could have been was 75. She left the exam feeling depressed and confused. She knew the information, but she never finished the test. Where did she go wrong?

Matthew's error was in test preparation. He studied the wrong material. Lisa's error was in test-taking strategies. She didn't know how to budget her time. Both these students need to learn how to assess their test-taking skills so that they can improve their grades.

Most students need to improve their test-taking strategies. They must examine the way they prepare for tests and take tests. Assessing test preparation and test-taking strategies is the beginning of improving test-taking skills.

Strategies for Preparing for the Test

1. Find out what to study.
   - Ask what material will be covered from your textbooks, class lectures, and notes.
   - Ask whether the test will be essay or objective.
2. Get organized for study.
   - Make sure that you budget enough study time in your schedule.
   - Summarize or outline the main points from your textbook and class notes.
   - Make sure that your assignments and notes are complete.
3. Study for the test.
   - Review your outline and summaries.
   - Answer end-of-chapter questions and old tests.
   - Design practice tests. Answer and correct your work.

Example 15–1

Matthew examined the test preparation strategies to see where he had made his mistake. He realized that he had never checked which material would be tested. He also had neglected to fill in notes from class lectures he missed. He had spent several hours preparing for his exam, but he had studied the wrong material.

Directions: Read over Strategies for Preparing for the Test. Assess your test preparation strategies. Which strategies could you improve?

EXERCISE
15–2

_____

_____

_____

_____

_____

_____

Strategies for Taking the Test

1. Follow directions carefully. Pay attention to the time limit and to the number of questions you are required to answer.
2. Read the entire test before you begin.
3. Answer the questions you know best first.

4. Be sure you answer the question asked. For example, if you are asked to *compare,* don't just give a *list.*

5. Budget your test-taking time. Do not spend too much time on one question.

6. Check your paper before you hand in your test to make sure that you have followed directions and that you have completely answered the questions.

Example 15–2

Lisa prepared for the test correctly, but she didn't know how to take the test. She didn't *budget her time.* She spent half the test time on one question, so she was unable to finish the test. Her low grade did not reflect her knowledge of the material, it indicated that she needed to improve her test-taking strategies.

EXERCISE 15–3

Directions: Read over Strategies for Taking the Test. Assess your test-taking strategies. Which strategies could you improve?

_____

_____

_____

_____

_____

_____

_____

_____

_____

▼ INTERPRETING ASSESSING YOUR TEST-TAKING SKILLS

Mindy asked her instructor whether the questions on her nutrition exam would be objective or essay. She knew which test chapters and class lectures would be included on the test. She began her preparation with two important steps:

1. The type of test
2. The material to be studied

She now had to decide how to use these two steps to prepare for her exam. She looked over the chapter titles in the text and reviewed the lecture headings in her notes. She didn't know whether she should first study the text and then study the notes or whether she should try to organize the material from both the text and the notes under topic headings.

Example 15–3

Text
Chapter 1 Nutrition calories
Chapter 2 Nutrition guidelines
Chapter 3 Nutrition for the elderly

Notes
Lecture 1 Calories and fat calories
Lecture 2 Menu planning for the home health care client
Lecture 3 The food groups
Lecture 4 Weight reduction
Lecture 5 Calories vs. fat content

Mindy decided to combine the information from both the text and lectures into categories so that she could better understand the information. *Categorizing* facts is a valuable study strategy. Therefore Mindy organized the material to be tested in the following pattern.

Nutrition Guidelines
The food groups
Menu planning for the home health care client
Nutrition for the elderly
Weight reduction
Nutrition calories
Calories and fat calories
Calories vs. fat content

By categorizing the material to be studied, Mindy has already analyzed the different assignments and organized them so she can improve her comprehension of the material.

Directions: Select one subject and organize the material to be studied for the next test in that subject.

EXERCISE 15–4

List the text chapters to be learned:

_____

_____

_____

_____

_____

_____

_____

List the lecture topics to be learned:

_____

_____

_____

_____

_____

_____

Categorize the information so that you can best learn the material:

_____

_____

_____

_____

_____

_____

_____

▼ APPLYING ASSESSING YOUR TEST-TAKING SKILLS

Mindy learned that the test on nutrition would have objective questions. When she received the material, she prepared thoroughly for the test by designing an objective test on the information she studied. The questions were a combination of *multiple-choice, true-false, short-answer,* and *matching.* When she finished, she corrected her practice test and looked up the answers to any questions she missed.

When Mindy designed her practice test, she remembered the specific strategies that would improve her effectiveness in taking objective tests.

Strategies for Taking Objective Tests

- For objective tests, learn specific facts as well as main ideas. Find out whether you will lose points for guessing. If not, answer *every* question.
- Read the test directions carefully.
- Read every question completely before answering.
- Be aware of such words as *never, always, except,* and *all.* These words are usually too broad and often signal an incorrect answer.

- Finish the test. In a timed test, answer the questions that you are sure of first and then answer the more difficult questions.
- Budget your test-taking time. Don't spend too much time on one question.
- Make sure that you fill in all the blanks in short-answer questions.
- When you answer matching questions, check off each answer as you make your match.
- In a true-false question, the answer choice must be totally true for you to select true as your answer.
- Check that you have lined up answers next to the correct questions before you hand in your paper.

Example 15–4

Some of Mindy's sample objective test questions were:

1. True or false
   Fat content alone is responsible for weight gain.
2. Steak is an example of a food that is _____.
   a. high in fat
   b. low fat
   c. nonfat
   d. unknown fat content
3. For a balanced diet, the menu should be planned around _____ essential food groups.
4. Matching

   _____ 1. complex carbohydrates   a. butter
   _____ 2. fat   b. meat
   _____ 3. protein   c. doughnuts
   _____ 4. simple carbohydrates   d. water
   _____ 5. fluid   e. cereal

Directions: Create an objective test for the test material you categorized. Use the four types of objective questions: short-answer, multiple-choice, true-false, and matching. Keep the objective test-taking strategies in mind as you design and take the test. Answer your questions and correct your answers.

EXERCISE
15–5

_____

_____

_____

_____

_____

_____

_____

_____

_____

_____

_____

_____

_____

_____

Alan was also taking an exam in nutrition. However, his instructor said that the exam would be essay. He received his test outlines and lecture notes and created essay questions based on the information. He then answered his practice questions and checked his answers for accuracy and organization. Alan applied the strategies that would improve his effectiveness in taking essay tests when he created his test questions and answers.

Strategies For Taking Essay Tests

- Read the directions carefully.
- Read all the test questions.
- Pay attention to the point value of each question, and budget your test time accordingly.
- Read the questions carefully and answer the question that is asked. Are you asked to _compare, list, classify,_ or _sequence_ information?
- Allow planning time for organizing your thoughts and writing an outline.

While writing your answer:

- State the main ideas clearly.
- Choose details that support the main idea.
- Write a logical conclusion.

After writing your answer:

- Check your answers for accuracy, organization, and completeness.

Example 15–5

Some of Alan's sample practice essay questions follow:

1. List the essential food groups needed in a daily diet.
2. Which is more effective for losing weight—counting fat or counting calories?
3. How does nutrition planning for the elderly differ from nutrition planning for the general population?

Directions: Create essay questions for the test material you categorized. Use the ideas presented in Strategies for Taking Essay Tests when you design and answer your essay questions.

EXERCISE **15–6**

_____

_____

_____

_____

_____

_____

▼ EVALUATING ASSESSING YOUR TEST-TAKING SKILLS

There are two times for you to evaluate your test-taking skills:

1. When you have finished preparing for the test
2. When you have received your test grade

Barry thought he was well prepared to take his exam in emergency medical care techniques. He reviewed the test chapters and the lecture notes. He designed his own practice test and gave himself a good score. He thought he would receive an A grade on the exam.

When his paper was returned, he had received a B–. He then had to evaluate his test-taking strategies and decided how he could improve his test-taking skills.

Example 15–6

Barry's Test Preparation. What went wrong? Barry studied his text chapters and lecture notes, but he neglected to underline all the main ideas in the text chapters. He also missed one lecture and forgot to ask someone in class about the topics covered during that lecture. Therefore, although Barry organized the material to be studied, he was working with incomplete information from the text and lectures.

By evaluating his work and assessing his test-taking strategies, Barry can now try to improve his work on the next exam rather than repeat the same mistake.

Directions: Evaluate your test preparation and test-taking strategies. Assess your work and decide how you can improve your test-taking skills.

EXERCISE **15–7**

_____

_____

_____

_____

_____

_____

_____

_____

CRITICAL READING

Previewing

Preview this selection. Think about what you already know about this topic. In the space provided, write what you still wish to know.

_____

_____

_____

_____

_____

_____

Questioning

Based on your preview, formulate questions that will help you learn what you still wish to know about the topic.

_____

_____

_____

_____

_____

_____

Reading

Read the following selection from *Saunders Fundamentals for Nursing Assistants* (Polaski and Warner, pp. 544-545):

Caring Comment

The nurse tells you if the patient needs to be weighed every day. You may hear the term "daily weights" used to refer to the order that the patient be weighed every day. If the patient is to be weighed daily, take the measurement at the same time every day and use the same scale. The patient should be dressed in similar clothes for each measurement. Ask the patient to void before the measurement is taken.

Obesity

One of the most common disruptions in nutrition is **obesity.** The person who is obese carries an accumulation of fat in the body. Obesity is an increase in weight above what is recommended for the individual's height and body build. The percentage of increase above normal determines whether a person is overweight, obese, or grossly obese.

OBESITY
overweight; the presence of too much fat in the body

- **Overweight**—10% above recommended weight
- **Obese**—15% above recommended weight
- **Grossly obese**—20% or more above recommended weight

Causes of Obesity

Excessive Intake. The amount of food or fluids taken in is more than the body needs to function. Often the intake consists of high-calorie and high-fat foods and fluids.

Lack of Exercise. The body needs exercise to burn off calories. The best exercise is walking. To be effective, exercise must be done three or four times a week for 20 - 30 minutes.

Disease that Affects Metabolism. In certain diseases such as hypothyroidism, obesity may occur despite a proper diet and adequate exercise.

Disruptions of Body Functioning Caused by Obesity

The person who is obese may experience the following disruptions in body functioning:

- Stress on the heart and lungs; these organs must work harder to circulate body fluids to the added cells
- **Hypertension**
- Inability to tolerate activity due to shortness of breath
- Stress on the pancreas, which produces insulin (in some people, this results in diabetes mellitus)

HYPERTENSION
persistent high blood pressure.

Care of the Obese Patient

The person who is overweight should be under the care and supervision of a health care professional. The health care professional recommends diet and exercises for the individual. You can help by providing support and encouragement to the patient.

Anorexia

Causes

Another disruption in nutrition is **anorexia.** Anorexia can be caused by diseases (such as cancer), certain medications that affect gastrointestinal functioning, or psychological factors. Because a daily intake of foods and fluids is needed to maintain a healthy body, the physician tries to discover cause of the anorexia.

Recording the Anorexic Patient's Intake

You may be asked to record the amount of food taken in by the anorexic patient using terms such as *good, fair,* or *poor.* Check your institution's guidelines when asked to use these words to describe intake. A scale such as the following may be used:

- Good—The patient ate 75% or more of the meal.
- Fair—The patient ate 50% of the meal.
- Poor—The patient ate less than 50% of the meal.

You may also want to record the specific amounts of food and fluids the anorexic patient has eaten. For example,

Half of a tuna salad sandwich
Half of a bowl of chicken soup
Two cups of black coffee
One cup of pudding
Half of a cup of pureed carrots

Care of the Anorexic Patient

The anorexic patient may be fatigued (tired) and uninterested in food or fluid. You have the following responsibilities in the care of the anorexic patient:

- Make mealtime pleasant. Place the patient in a sitting position if allowed. Help the patient with toileting before mealtime. Do not hurry when you take the meal into the room.
- Check the environment. Make sure no noxious (foul) odors are present when the meal is served.
- Provide support. Eating is a social activity, so your presence may encourage a patient to eat more.
- Provide the prescribed diet. The nurse tells you the diet that has been ordered for the patient. Match the diet slip with the patient's identification bracelet to be certain you are giving the correct diet to the patient.
- Provide small amounts of food or fluid frequently. A patient may be able to tolerate small amounts offered often better than large amounts of food offered infrequently.
- Weigh the patient daily. A record of daily weight measurements shows when the patient gains weight.

Alternate Routes for Feeding: The patient may require tube feedings through a tube inserted into the stomach or through a special tube inserted into a vein (hyperalimentation). The nurse is responsible for these alternate feedings.

Applying

In the space provided, answer your questions.

_____

_____

_____

_____

_____

_____

Evaluating

Were you able to answer all your questions? Yes _____ No _____. Did the selection give you enough information about the topic? Explain.

_____

_____

_____

_____

_____

_____

Check the accuracy of your answers by finding the specific information in the selection.

STUDENT JOURNAL

List what you have learned about assessing your test-taking skills.	How would you apply this knowledge to your study or work in the health fields?

References

Beaver BV: Feline Behavior: A Guide for Veterinarians. Philadelphia, W.B. Saunders, 1992.

Bonewit-West K: Computer Concepts and Applications for the Medical Office. Philadelphia, W.B. Saunders, 1993.

Chabner D-E: The Language of Medicine, 4th ed. Philadelphia, W.B. Saunders, 1991.

Diehl MO, Fordney MT: Medical Typing and Transcribing: Techniques and Procedures, 3rd ed. Philadelphia, W.B. Saunders, 1991.

Flynn JC Jr (Ed.): Procedures in Phlebotomy. Philadelphia, W.B. Saunders, 1994.

Henry MC, Stapleton ER (Eds.): EMT Prehospital Care. Philadelphia, W.B. Saunders, 1992.

Kinn ME, Woods MA, Derge EF: The Medical Assistant: Administrative and Clinical, 7th ed. Philadelphia, W.B. Saunders, 1993.

LaFleur-Brooks M (Ed.): Health Unit Coordinating, 3rd ed. Philadelphia, W.B. Saunders, 1993.

McCurnin DM (Ed.): Clinical Textbook for Veterinary Technicians, 3rd ed. Philadelphia, W.B. Saunders, 1994.

Polaski A, Warner JP: Saunders Fundamentals for Nursing Assistants. Philadelphia, W.B. Saunders, 1994.

Solomon EP: Introduction to Human Anatomy and Physiology. Philadelphia, W.B. Saunders, 1992.

Answer Key

CHAPTER 1

EXERCISE 1–1

Answers will vary.

EXERCISE 1–2

1. pertaining to the skull
2. pertaining to the hip bone
3. muscle separating the abdominal and the thoracic cavities
4. backbone
5. voice box
6. throat
7. flexible connective tissue attached to bones at joints
8. windpipe
9. regions of DNA within each chromosome
10. the total of the chemical processes in a cell

EXERCISE 1–3

1. high blood pressure
2. overactive thyroid
3. under the skin
4. doctor who treats diseases in urinary tract
5. study of the blood
6. foreknowledge
7. study of nerves
8. process of cutting back
9. study of woman and female disorders
10. to cut into

EXERCISE 1–4

1. chronic, recurrent dermatosis marked by itchy, scaly, red patches carved by silvery scales
2. Psoralen–ultraviolet A light therapy
3. Answers will vary.

EXERCISE 1–5

1. *in vitro:* in the test tube
   in vivo: in the body
2. with the radiation given off by the radionuclide
3. A specific radionuclide is incorporated into a chemical substance and administered to a patient.
4. to detect hormones and drugs in a patient's blood; to monitor the amount of digitalis, a drug used to treat heart disease; in a patient's bloodstream; and to detect hypothyroidism in newborn infants
5. These procedures give physicians a way to detect hormones, drugs, and radioactive substances in the body.

EXERCISE 1–6

1. user passwords
2. place of services
3. the physicians in your medical practice

4. to process insurance claims
5. You would make errors on bills and insurance forms and have to waste time correcting your work.

EXERCISE 1–7

1. lack of oxygen flow to the brain evidenced by no pulse and respirations
2. a state of sustained oxygen deprivation after which recovery without brain damage is unlikely
3. Answers will vary.

CRITICAL READING

Answers will vary.

STUDENT JOURNAL

Answers will vary.

CHAPTER 2

EXERCISE 2–1

Answers will vary.

EXERCISE 2–2

1. O
2. F
3. F
4. O
5. F
6. O
7. O
8. F
9. O
10. F

EXERCISE 2–3

Examples may vary.
1. falls   Falls may result in broken bones.
2. burns   Hot food or fluid can result in serious burns.
3. suffocation   Suffocation occurs when an object does not allow air to enter the lungs.
4. aspiration   A small object when breathed into the lungs may block the air passages.
5. poisoning   Harmful fluids could result in accidental poisoning.
6. motor vehicle accidents   The law in many states requires the use of safety car seats for infants, toddlers, and young children.

EXERCISE 2–4

Answers may vary, but a possible answer would be:

1. Sports injuries cause accidental falls.
2. Children between 6 and 12 may get burned by playing with matches.
3. Unsupervised water play leads to drowning.
4. Children run out in traffic.
5. Unfamiliar people could be a source of danger.

EXERCISE 2–5

Answers will vary.

EXERCISE 2–6

Answers will vary.

CRITICAL READING

Answers will vary.

STUDENT JOURNAL

Answers will vary.

CHAPTER 3

EXERCISE 3–1

Answers will vary.

EXERCISE 3–2

1. P N
2. P N
3. N P
4. P N
5. P N
6. N P
7. P N
8. N P
9. N P
10. P N

EXERCISE 3–3

Answers will vary.

EXERCISE 3–4

Answers will vary.

EXERCISE 3–5

Answers will vary.

EXERCISE 3–6

Answers will vary.

EXERCISE 3–7

Answers will vary.

CRITICAL READING

Answers will vary.

STUDENT JOURNAL

Answers will vary.

CHAPTER 4

EXERCISE 4–1

Answers will vary.

EXERCISE 4–2

1. Negative: emergency road, victims, devastating, accident
2. Objective
3. Negative: monitored, rising
4. Objective
5. Negative: lessen, discomfort, painkillers
6. Objective
7. Positive: relieved
8. Positive: comfortable, flattering
9. Objective
10. Negative: obese, ordered, 80

EXERCISE 4–3

1. startling results, experts, no time
2. Margorie reacted to the positive feeling generated by these emotionally charged words and did not carefully examine the facts before she made her judgment.
3. nutritional value, appropriate length of time to reach target weight

EXERCISE 4–4

Answers will vary.
Possible Answer: No, this was not a satisfactory weight loss program. There was not enough variety (no protein) or enough substance, and the diet was too extreme. Adhering to this diet would be difficult.

EXERCISE 4–5

Answers will vary.
Possible Answers:
1. meat, fish, nuts
2. nuts, peanut butter, dry beans
3. milk, cheese, ice cream, yogurt
4. important bone growth

EXERCISE 4–6

Answers will vary.

EXERCISE 4–7

1. grain, cereal, fruit and vegetables
2. doughnuts, potato chips, etc

EXERCISE 4–8

Answers will vary.

EXERCISE 4–9

1. vitamins C and B
2. Water carries important substances to the cell and takes away the waste products produced by the cell.
3. Carbohydrates are a source of energy in the body.
4. Too much cholesterol can block arteries.
5. Eat a varied diet chosen from the five food groups.

EXERCISE 4–10

Cereal: Cereal is a complex carbohydrate; a doughnut is a simple carbohydrate. Complex carbohydrates take longer for the body to break down and use and a person does not feel hunger as quickly.

EXERCISE 4–11

Answers will vary.

CRITICAL READING

Answers will vary.

STUDENT JOURNAL

Answers will vary.

CHAPTER 5

EXERCISE 5–1

Answers will vary.

EXERCISE 5–2

Answers will vary.

EXERCISE 5–3

Answers will vary.

EXERCISE 5–4

Answers will vary.

EXERCISE 5–5

Answers will vary.

EXERCISE 5–6

Answers will vary.

EXERCISE 5–7

Answers will vary.

CRITICAL READING

Answers will vary.

STUDENT JOURNAL

Answers will vary.

CHAPTER 6

EXERCISE 6–1

Answers will vary.

EXERCISE 6–2

1. sequence
2. comparison and contrast
3. classification
4. sequence
5. examples and illustration
6. cause and effect
7. sequence
8. problem solving

9. comparison and contrast
10. cause and effect

EXERCISE 6–3

1. detail 4
2. detail 4
3. details 4 and 5
4. detail 3
5. detail 1

EXERCISE 6–4

Answers will vary.

EXERCISE 6–5

Answers will vary.

CRITICAL READING

Answers will vary.

STUDENT JOURNAL

Answers will vary.

CHAPTER 7

EXERCISE 7–1

Answers will vary.

EXERCISE 7–2

Answers will vary but should contain the following point: Summary writing teaches you to ensure that you understand the written article so that you can substitute the author's words for your own and find the main ideas.

EXERCISE 7–3

1. *Time order summary:* To show in what order important ideas occurred in the article to be summarized
2. *Visual mapping summary:* To show the important details that relate to certain main ideas in the article to be summarized
3. *Summary chart:* To show the more complex relationships among important ideas in the article to be summarized, that is, cause and effect, comparison and contrast, and problem solving.

Exercise 7–4

Heading Question: What is the liver's unusual circulation? Eliminate the following:
Paragraph 1: The first four sentences.
Paragraph 2: Nutrients are absorbed into these capillaries.
Paragraph 3: The first sentence.

Exercise 7–5

Eliminate the following: For instance, the Pathology Department . . . medicolegal reports are usually done in the private medical office.

Exercise 7–6

Answers will vary but should resemble the following:

Unimportant Ideas
1. through autopsies much knowledge . . . treatment of disease
2. includes a description . . . that govern autopsies
3. an autopsy may be ordered . . . the cause of death
4. pathologist, forensic pathologist . . . and psychologist

Repetitive Ideas
1. A visual and microscopic examination . . . and related structures
2. (such as violent death, . . . and so forth)
3. (in story form)
4. (by the numbers)
5. (hand drawings or anatomical forms)
6. which is a brief resume . . . prior to demise
7. (visual examination of the organs . . . and examination)
8. (an examination of the particular organs . . . microscope)
9. (or final pathological diagnosis . . . after its termination)

Clusters
1. Written report done in any of the following ways:
   a. narrative
   b. pictorial
   c. sentence completion
   d. multiple choice
   e. problem oriented

2. Clinical history of hospital stay:
   a. pathological diagnosis
   b. results of gross anatomy findings
   c. results of microscopic exam
   d. epicrisis
3. Permission from next of kin
   a. must become part of record in 90 days
   b. must be obtained for organ removal
   c. must be obtained for victims of crimes
   d. must be obtained for unattached people
   e. may involve different medical professionals

Exercise 7–7

Answers will vary.

Exercise 7–8

Answers will vary.

Exercise 7–9

Answers will vary.

Exercise 7–10

Answers will vary.

Critical Reading

Answers will vary.

Student Journal

Answers will vary.

CHAPTER 8

Exercise 8–1

Answers will vary.

Exercise 8–2

Inductive reasoning = Specific → General

Exercise 8–3

Answers will vary but should include the idea of reasoning from the general to the specific.

Exercise 8–4

Answers will vary, but steps 3 and 4 should resemble the examples given in Figures 8–1 and 8–2.

Exercise 8–5

Answers will vary.

EXERCISE 8–6

Answers will vary.

EXERCISE 8–7

1. I
2. I
3. D
4. D
5. I
6. I
7. D
8. D
9. D
10. I

CRITICAL READING

Answers will vary.

STUDENT JOURNAL

Answers will vary.

CHAPTER 9

EXERCISE 9–1

Answers will vary.

EXERCISE 9–2

1. Fallacy—cross out
2. OK
3. Fallacy—cross out
4. OK
5. Fallacy—cross out
6. Fallacy—cross out
7. OK
8. OK
9. Fallacy—cross out
10. OK

EXERCISE 9–3

1. c, e
2. e, c
3. c, e
4. e, c
5. c, e
6. e, c
7. e, c
8. c, e
9. e, c
10. c, e

EXERCISE 9–4

Answers will vary but should include these general ideas:

1. I did well in high school math. I will work as hard as I did in high school to do as well in college math.
2. Since she has a talent for training her own pets, she may be good at training other animals.
3. I cannot assume that my state doesn't have homeless people just because my town doesn't have homeless people.
4. If the 10-year-old patient keeps taking care of his teeth all his adult life, he may never have any cavities.
5. I cannot assume that the doctor will be late this time. I will call ahead of time to see how long I must wait.

EXERCISE 9–5

It is beneficial for the federal . . . for the government to do so—CR
Elderly and chronically ill—C
Many millions of dollars will be saved—E
Thus, if all elderly . . . money would be saved—Jump
It is a wise idea . . . smart to do so—CR
Because of home health care—C
The patient can persevere.—E
They are more comfortable—E
By remaining in familiar—C
Patients are more content—E
They are not isolated—C
Home health care is helpful . . . in many ways—CR
Consequently, patients with pulmonary . . . institutionalization—Jump
Home care is desired . . . their loved ones—CR

EXERCISE 9–6

Answers will vary but should resemble this format:

It is beneficial for the federal and state governments to financially support home health care workers because it is a financially responsible position to take. Many millions of dollars will be saved if the elderly and chronically ill can be kept out of hos-

pitals and nursing homes. At present, it costs $180,000 annually to maintain an elderly person in a nursing home. This same patient can be cared for at home with a daily full time home health care worker for $30,000. Thus, *when the situation is appropriate, many elderly patients can be cared for at home.*

It is a wise idea to support the home health care project any way we can because *some patients can gain by home health care.* Because of home health care, the patients can persevere in much of their regular daily routine. They are more comfortable, physically, when they remain in familiar surroundings. Patients are more content emotionally because they are not isolated from family and friends. Home health care is helpful for patients because it helps people *maintain their lifestyle.*

One example of good home health care concerned 80 year old Maimie. She was diagnosed as suffering from chronic bronchitis and asthma. It was becoming increasingly more difficult for Maimie to live independently. Her family considered either a nursing home or home health care for her. After considering both the costs and Maimie's emotional well-being, the family decided on home health care. A worker now visits her four days a week and helps with bathing, shopping, housekeeping, and minor medical procedures. Maimie is still able to visit with her friends and family and on good days go out to restaurants, movies, and card games. Consequently, *when appropriate, some patients with* pulmonary problems would do better with home health care than with institutionalization. Home care is desired by more patients and their families because it is *relatively cheaper than institutionalization and may keep patients independent longer.*

EXERCISE 9–7

Answers will vary.

CRITICAL READING

Answers will vary.

STUDENT JOURNAL

Answers will vary.

CHAPTER 10

EXERCISE 10–1

Answers will vary.

EXERCISE 10–2

Answers will vary.

EXERCISE 10–3

1. kilometer
2. meter
3. liter
4. metric ton
5. meter
6. gram
7. square kilometer
8. square centimeter
9. kilogram
10. square meter

EXERCISE 10–4

1. 0.45 kilogram
2. 2.2 pounds
3. 3.28 feet
4. 0.3 meter
5. 0.04 ounce
6. 28.35 grams
7. 1.61 kilograms
8. 0.62 mile
9. 0.155 square inch
10. 6.45 square centimeters

EXERCISE 10–5

1. a. 0.4
   b. 0.24
   c. 0.12
   d. 0.88
   e. 1.92
2. a. 14.4
   b. 38.4
   c. 70.8
   d. 104.4
   e. 126
3. a. 6.4
   b. 11.6
   c. 26.4
   d. 71.2
   e. 128.4
4. a. 4.55
   b. 51.87
   c. 179.27
   d. 257.53
   e. 502.32
5. a. 17.1
   b. 35.15
   c. 259.35

d. 607.05

e. 1663.45

EXERCISE 10–6

1. 31.76 ounces
2. 18.16 ounces
3. 13.6 ounces
4. Car 2, 3.58 miles
5. 38.8 inches
6. 2413 millimeters
7. 362,600,000 square kilometers
8. 4.4 inches
9. 348 feet
10. 9.1 meters
11. 14.4 meters
12. Nurse Clinton, 5.4 meters
13. 25.44 quarts
14. 72 square meters
15. 1 ounce
16. 8.89 centimeters
17. 215.6 pounds
18. 2.275 metric tons
19. 32.28 square feet
20. 708.66 inches

EXERCISE 10–7

Answers will vary.

CRITICAL READING

Answers will vary.

STUDENT JOURNAL

Answers will vary.

CHAPTER 11

EXERCISE 11–1

Answers will vary.

EXERCISE 11–2

1. a. figure out
   b. each
   c. division
   d. 1
   e. 22
2. a. figure out
   b. total
   c. addition

d. 1

e. 15 + 5 = 20 miles

3. a. a midpoint
   b. average
   c. division
   d. 2
   e. tied (1 in 3)
4. a. approximate
   b. total, hourly
   c. addition and division
   d. 2
   e. $20 per hour
5. a. subtract
   b. deduct
   c. subtraction
   d. 1
   e. $99.95

EXERCISE 11–3

1. a. 10 servings minestrone = 175 calories
   6 servings vegetable soup = 180 calories
   b. Because the number of servings and the total calories are the important facts needed.
   minestrone soup: $^{10}/_{175}$ = $17\,^1/_2$ calories per serving
   vegetable soup: $^6/_{180}$ = 30 calories per serving
   c. The vegetable soup has more calories per serving.
2. a. half order at $6.98
   1 order at $3.95
   b. Because $^1/_2$ has to be compared to 1 to answer problem
   $^1/_2$ (6.98) = 3.49
   1 (3.95) = 3.95
   c. Marian paid more for dinner.
3. a. 425
   450
   %
   b. Because percent of numbers is needed in solution
   c. There is a 6% difference in the calories.
4. a. $2\,^1/_2$ miles before work
   $3\,^1/_4$ miles after work
   b. Because solution called for total mileage
   c. $5\,^3/_4$ miles (5.75 miles)
5. a. TV cost $250
   VCR cost $219
   b. Because needed for total

a. TV-VCR combination cost $438
b. Because needed for comparison
c. Yes. Combination is better value: $438 compared to $469

Exercise 11–4

1. $2\frac{1}{4}$ hours
   $^{90}/_{40} = ^{9}/_{4} = 2.25$ hours
   you can estimate the travel time
2. 15 pounds
   calculate total weight loss
3. Employee B by 20 units
   could measure efficiency of each worker
4. 1.38
   $^{22}/_{1.75} = 12.57$ calories per ounce; $^{54}/_{2} = 27$ calories per ounce.
   information needed to plan for a lower calorie dressing
   Solution: cucumber yogurt
5. 82
   $\dfrac{(72 + 85 + 78 + 93)}{4} = \dfrac{328}{4} = 82$
   determining an average helps you to estimate a semester grade

Exercise 11–5

1. Approximately 2 pounds
   $^{35}/_{16}$ rounds to 2
2. 16 cookies
   1 dozen converted to 12, multiplied by 2 is 24; $^{3}/_{3} - ^{1}/_{3} = ^{2}/_{3}$; $^{2}/_{3}$ of 24 cookies = 16
3. $1\frac{7}{8}$ miles
   $^{3}/_{4} \times ^{5}/_{2} = ^{15}/_{8} = 1\frac{7}{8}$
   I multiplied fractions to get the answer.
4. 6.4 ounces
   $^{8}/_{5} = 1.6$ $1.6 \times 4 = 6.4$ ounces
   I divided the total weight by the sum of the ratio. I then multiplied the quotient by the meat part of the ratio.
5. $70
   Multiply the cost of the sweater by 2.

Critical Reading

Answers will vary.

Student Journal

Answers will vary.

CHAPTER 12

Exercise 12–1

Answers will vary.

Exercise 12–2

1. division and multiplication, $^{20}/_{1750} \times 4 = \$350$
2. multiplication, $0.98 \times 12 = \$11.76$
3. multiplication and division, 4 meters $\times$ 100 = 400 centimeters, $^{400}/_{12} = 33\frac{1}{3}$ centimeters
4. addition, 7 PM
5. multiplication and subtraction, $2 \times 7 = 14$ days; $23 - 14 = 9$ days late

Exercise 12–3

Facts Needed	Answer
1. a	$2
2. a, b	10%
3. b, c	7.5 L
4. a, b, c	75%
5. b, c	40 minutes

Exercise 12–4

1. $^{160}/_{30} = 5.3$. Each employee should be assigned five packages a year.
2. $1000 \times 300 = 300{,}000$ sq. feet; $300{,}000 \times 0.30 = 90{,}000$; $300{,}000 \times 0.25 = 75{,}000$; $90{,}000 - 75{,}000 = 15{,}000$
3. $\$8.50 + \$1.50 = \$10$; $\$10 - \$6 = \$4$; $\$4 \times \$40 = \$160 \times 2 = \$320$
4. 0.5 km
5. $^{35}/_{75} = ^{7}/_{15}$; $^{7}/_{15} = 46.6\%$ or $46\frac{2}{3}\%$

Exercise 12–5

1. Answers will vary.
2. Answers will vary.
3. Answers will vary.
4. Answers will vary.
5. Answers will vary.

Critical Reading

Answers will vary.

Student Journal

Answers will vary.

CHAPTER 13

Exercise 13–1

Answers will vary.

EXERCISE 13–2

Answers will vary.

EXERCISE 13–3

Answers will vary.

EXERCISE 13–4

Answers will vary.

EXERCISE 13–5

Answers will vary.

EXERCISE 13–6

Answers will vary.

EXERCISE 13–7

Answers will vary.

EXERCISE 13–8

1. Look up terms in a dictionary or glossary.
2. Reread the passage, aloud if necessary.
3. Check in an encyclopedia or easier text.
4. Rewrite or summarize the circulation pattern in your own words.
5. Check the term in a medical dictionary.
6. Consult with an easier text.
7. Reread the page aloud.
8. Rewrite the process in your own words.
9. Look up the terms in a medical dictionary.
10. Read an easier text or look up spirometric equipment in an encyclopedia.

EXERCISE 13–9

Answers will vary.

EXERCISE 13–10

Answers will vary.

CRITICAL READING

Answers will vary.

STUDENT JOURNAL

Answers will vary.

CHAPTER 14

EXERCISE 14–1

Answers will vary.

EXERCISE 14–2

Answers will vary.

EXERCISE 14–3

1. section 3
2. section 1
3. section 5
4. section 4
5. section 2
6. section 1
7. section 3
8. section 5
9. section 2
10. section 4

EXERCISE 14–4

Answers will vary.

EXERCISE 14–5

Answers will vary.

EXERCISE 14–6

Answers will vary.

CRITICAL READING

Answers will vary.

STUDENT JOURNAL

Answers will vary.

CHAPTER 15

EXERCISE 15–1

Answers will vary.

EXERCISE 15–2

Answers will vary.

EXERCISE 15–3

Answers will vary.

EXERCISE 15–4

Answers will vary.

EXERCISE 15–5

Answers will vary.

Exercise 15–6

Answers will vary.

Critical Reading

Answers will vary.

Exercise 15–7

Answers will vary.

Student Journal

Answers will vary.

Index

Note: Page numbers in *italics* refer to reading selections.